Healing with Handmade Bread

Healing with Handmade Bread

From Start to Finish in Just Two Hours

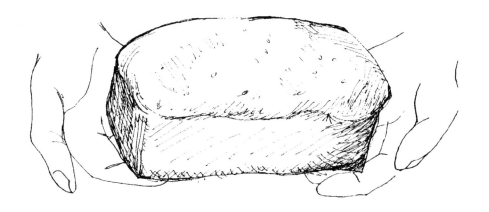

Learn to Make Bread as You Heal from Breast Cancer

Kathy Summers

*illustrated by
Sarah Corry*

iUniverse, Inc.
New York Lincoln Shanghai

Healing with Handmade Bread
From Start to Finish in Just Two Hours

All Rights Reserved © 2004 by Kathy Summers

No part of this book may be reproduced or transmitted in any form or by any means, graphic, electronic, or mechanical, including photocopying, recording, taping, or by any information storage retrieval system, without the written permission of the publisher.

iUniverse, Inc.

For information address:
iUniverse, Inc.
2021 Pine Lake Road, Suite 100
Lincoln, NE 68512
www.iuniverse.com

ISBN: 0-595-30451-6

Printed in the United States of America

For Lily and Earl

Many Thanks

to my husband, who 36 years ago suggested I make bread from scratch,

to our children and our grandchildren, who grew eating our handmade bread and learned to make bread themselves,

to my loving parents,

to all those who have enjoyed eating our bread these many years,

to Dr. Mari Nakashizuka for her kind and excellent care,

to my dear friends Pat and Nancy,

to Hob,

to the Healing Touch/Bosom Buddies community in Hawaii that helped me with my breast cancer,

to the American Cancer Society's program, Reach to Recovery,

to Denise,

to Mary,

to Sarah,

to the kind, helpful people at iUniverse

and to God for all things.

Contents

Introduction 1

Breast Cancer 3

My Diagnosis and Treatment 5

Tips for Breast Cancer Patients 7

My Breast Cancer Journal 13

Equipment 25

Ingredients 29
    Leaven 30
    Liquids 31
    Wheat Flour 31
    Other Grain Flour, Flakes and Cereal 32
    Non-grain Flour and Flakes 32
    Salt 33
    Sweetener 33
    Fat 33
    Eggs 34
    Spices 34
    Extracts 34
    Nuts 34
    Seeds 34
    Cheese 34
    Fresh Fruit 35
    Fresh Vegetables 35
    Canned Fruit and Vegetables 35
    Dried Fruit 35

Techniques 37
- Stay Focused 38
- Never Give Up 38
- Read the Recipe 38
- Quantity 38
- Prepare the Work Space 38
- Proof the Yeast 38
- Clean as You Work 39
- Grease 39
- Measure the Ingredients 39
- Mix 40
- Dust 40
- Preheat and Check Oven Accuracy 40
- Knead 40
- Too Busy to Shape the Dough Now 41
- Shape 41
- Rise 43
- Glaze 43
- Toppings 44
- Bake 44
- Cool 44
- Write Notes 45
- Slice 45
- Thank 45
- Share 45
- Store 45
- Freeze 46
- Defrost 46
- Practice 46

How to Use the Recipes 47

Invent Your Own Recipes 49

Use Other Recipes and Make Them This Simple Way 51

Things That Can Go Wrong and How to Fix Them 53

Recipes 55

Whole Grain Bread and Rolls 57
   Whole-wheat 58
   Milk/Wheat 60
   Buttermilk/Wheat 60
   Whole-wheat/Nut 61
   Whole-wheat/Sunflower Seed 61
   Wheat Germ 61
   Wheat Bran 61
   Cornmeal/Wheat 61
   Buckwheat 61
   Eight-grain Cereal 61
   Potato/Wheat 62
   100% Whole-wheat 63
   Multi-grain 65
   High Protein Multi-grain 68
   Seed 71
   Rye 74
   Oatmeal Raisin 77

White Bread and Rolls 81
   White 82
   Milk 84
   Buttermilk 84
   Soymilk 85
   Potato 85
   Cornmeal 85
   Oatmeal 85
   Wheat Germ 85
   Nutritious White 86

French Bread and Rolls 89
   French 90
   Vienna 93
   Semolina French 93
   Whole-wheat French 93
   Olive 94
   Cornmeal French 94
   Rye French 94
   Multi-grain/Seed French 94

Sweet Bread **95**
    Challah 96
    Whole-wheat Challah 98
    Cinnamon 99
    Cinnamon/Raisin 101

Rolls **103**
    Italian 104
    Milk 106
    Buttermilk 106
    Whole-wheat 107
    Oat 107
    Cinnamon 108
    Cinnamon/Raisin 110
    Cinnamon/Apple 111
    Soft Pan 112
    Orange 114

Pretzels **115**
    Pretzels 116
    Whole-wheat 119
    Rye 119
    Cornmeal 119
    Semolina 119
    Buckwheat/Fennel 119
    Pizza/Feta Cheese 120
    Onion 120
    Garlic 120
    Everything 120
    Pumpkin/Date 120
    Sweet Potato/Cheddar 120
    Banana/Macadamia Nut 121
    Apple/Cinnamon 121

Special Bread **123**
    Bread Sticks 124
    Pizza Dough 127
    Focaccia 129
    Sun Dried Tomato Focaccia 131

Muffins	133
Tips for Excellent Muffins	135
Things that Can Go Wrong and How to Fix Them	137
Bluberry	138
Raisin/Nut	140
Date	140
Cheese	140
Corn	141
Corn/Bluberry	142
Corn/Cheese	142
Pumpkin	143
Banana	144
Applesauce	145
Bran	146
Gingerbread	148
Oatcakes	150
Glossary	153
Bibliography	157
Ordering Information	159

INTRODUCTION

Dear friends,

I have made handmade bread almost every day for the last thirty-six years. We raised a family of nine children and they are mostly made of handmade bread. Being so busy with our children, I had to figure out a way of making bread that was not only nutritious and delicious, but also fast and easy. I have taught our six daughters and hundreds of other people how to make bread. Many say it is the best bread they have ever eaten and the first time they have been successful making bread.

This book takes you carefully through the fundamental knowledge and steps of making bread. The instructions are simple and specific. The ingredients are rapidly mixed together. There is a short kneading time and no first rising of the dough. All the yeast bread recipes are made with instant yeast. The bread is mixed, kneaded, shaped, raised and then baked. Every recipe can be completed from start to finish within two hours.

As you stay focused on making the bread, your mind will quiet. Enjoy the peacefulness.

There are many whole grain recipes. There are traditional favorite recipes and recipes that you have not seen before.

First read all the instructional sections. Next read the recipe and make the basic recipe in each of the eight types of bread. Then move on to the variations and other recipes in each section. As you practice, making bread will become easy. You will have many fans enjoying your delicious bread.

Halfway through writing this book, I learned I had breast cancer. As I recovered, one of the first things I did was to make bread again. I realized as I made bread, how the use of my hands, arms and body were very therapeutic to my healing. I felt called by God to write this book a little differently.

I thought what a gift it would be if women with breast cancer learned the art of making handmade bread. It would help their physical, mental and spiritual healing. I have included some tips I learned dealing with breast cancer and some of my journal entries.

This is a book for everyone, not only women with breast cancer. Just as homemade bread is enjoyed by almost everyone, most people have either had cancer themselves or been close to someone else who has.

Welcome to the world of beautiful handmade bread: the feel, the smell, the taste, the quietness and the sharing. "Give us this day our daily bread."

With love and God's blessings,

Kathy

Breast Cancer

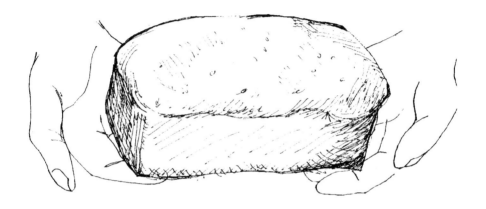

My Diagnosis and Treatment

I took estrogen for ten years after a hysterectomy and up through the time of my second lumpectomy. Then I stopped taking estrogen. I now think it is better to not take estrogen because of recent research, but this is something important to discuss with your doctor as you grow older.

Prior to my cancer, I had two other lumpectomies. In the first lumpectomy, the breast surgeon found lobular carcinoma in situ. She wanted me to take the medication Tamoxifen. I tried to take it, but I had difficult side effects, so I did not continue to take it. The second time I had a lumpectomy, she found hyperplasia tissue. Neither lobular carcinoma in situ or hyperplasia tissue are considered cancer, but they are serious warnings that cancer may come.

In my yearly mammogram last year, the radiologist found microcalcifications in my milk duct area. The biopsy was malignant. The diagnosis was ductal carcinoma in situ. There was no cancer in my lymph nodes. My treatment options were a lumpectomy to be done with the biopsy, followed by radiation, or to have a mastectomy. I chose to have a mastectomy. I did not need further treatment, so I have not experienced the removal of many lymph nodes, radiation or chemotherapy.

A breast surgeon checks me every three months. I am grateful I have been able to go to her, instead of a general surgeon, because she is aware of all the latest developments with breast cancer. I have seen her every three month for about five years.

TIPS FOR BREAST CANCER PATIENTS

There are many options in treatment for breast cancer and choosing what to do is often very difficult for people. Before choosing your treatment, talk to several knowledgeable people about your treatment options as doctors, nurses, and cancer patients.

Study breast cancer literature from the American Cancer Society. Read books about breast cancer. Look at breast cancer sites on the Internet. I recommend *Dr. Susan Love's Breast Book* by Dr. Susan Love. Some helpful sites on the Internet are: komen.org, cancersource.com, cancer.org. You can look at books on breast cancer on the Amazon.com web site. See which sound interesting to you and order them. Large bookstores always have books on breast cancer.

Prayer is a great help. A belief in a loving God and in eternal life helps to put things in perspective.

Have a spiritual practice at a church or with a group of people.

Learn to meditate. There are helpful groups that can teach you as well as useful books as: *The Miracle of Mindfulness* by Thich Nhat Hahn, *Full Catastrophe Living* and *Wherever You Go There You Are* by Jon Kabat-Zinn.

Study mindfulness. Be mindful of the present moment. Concentrate when you are listening to people, feel the ground and your legs when you walk, eat slowly and really taste the food, etc. Do not look back very often or try to look too far in the future. Live each day the best you can. It is the only day you have.

Learn to be at peace when you are alone. Being alone is very different than being lonely. If you believe in God, enjoy God's presence when you are alone. I believe God is always beside us, loving us. I believe angels are with us also.

Keep a journal for you, your loved ones and others. Journaling helps you to sort out what you are feeling.

Humor is always helpful. Find ways to laugh each day.

Learn to do relaxing breathing techniques such as the Relaxation Response. Many good books are available on breathing as: *The Relaxation Response* and *Beyond the Relaxation Response* by Herbert Benson. Relaxing breathing is a skill to develop. It takes practice for many weeks and then it will help you. Do not give up when you first try it.

Share what is happening to you and what you are feeling with your family, friends, doctors, nurses and technicians. It is very important not to keep your feelings or questions to yourself.

Be patient with family members. They are also affected by cancer. They will stop to help you, but their lives need to go on as normally as possible. Stay interested in what they are doing.

You will need friends as well as family. Sometimes family members have a hard time knowing that you are suffering. A kind friend can sometimes deal with it more easily.

Call the Reach for Recovery Program with the American Cancer Society. They will send a representative who has had a similar cancer to yours to help you. She will bring you a lot of information and other helpful items.

If you need more support, join a breast cancer support group. I did not join one, but I had many people to talk with and who cared about me. I was also already very familiar with breast cancer from being a hospice and Healing Touch volunteer. I knew a lot of what would happen already and how people react.

If you have a mastectomy, when the doctor says it is all right to do the suggested daily exercises with your arm, be consistent. The exercises will help restore the range of motion in your arm.

When you are able to exercise, do so each day for at least 20 minutes. Walk, do yoga stretches, work out at a YMCA gym or another gym that will help you to know how to use their exercise machines. When the incision is healed, go swimming. Exercise helps to chase away depression, give you strength and better health.

See a good counselor if you have depression.

Each day eat a variety of fruits, vegetables and whole grains. Eat healthful sources of protein. Drink plenty of good water.

Sleep as much as you need to. Go to bed early and get up early.

Give service to others. Even tiny acts of service will bless you and those you serve.

Be a good listener. Read excellent books on listening as: *The Art of Sacred Listening* by Kay Lindahl and *I Don't Have to Make Everything Better* by Gary and Joy Lundberg.

Listen to inspiring and uplifting music.

Read inspirational books as: *Pay Attention For Goodness Sake* by Sylvia Boornstein, and *Peace in Every Step* by Thich Nhat Hahn. Read books from you religious faith that will help you grow closer to God.

Get a massage sometimes from a good massage therapist.

Get family members or friends to massage your feet. When you can, massage theirs another time.

Look at beauty in nature. Enjoy flowers, trees, mountains, the ocean, etc.

When you feel better, take a trip with someone you love.

To Help Ease the Pain After a Mastectomy:

Massage the area directly or through a small pillow.

When it is appropriate, do not wear clothes over the surgical sight. Clothes can feel very painful when the nerves start working again.

Wear a stretchy, smooth camisole top under your clothes. Get three or four of them so you don't have to wash them so often. They will protect you so your clothes do not rub on the surgical site.

Rub a deep menthol ointment around, but not on the surgical area.

Use an ice pack on the area or gentle heat.

Learn to do Healing Touch on yourself and have someone else do it for you. Healing Touch "is a gentle placement of hands on and around the body. The goal is to restore balance to the mind, body and spirit and encourage the body to heal itself." See www.healingtouch.net.

Remember that the pain will come and go.

Put an antibiotic ointment on the incision if it gets red and irritated

Supplements that I Take Now to Help Prevent Further Cancer:

a multi-vitamin that contains selenium, vitamin E and the B vitamins.
vitamin C
calcium
magnesium
co-enzyme Q-10

Before taking any supplements, consult your doctor and do research. There is a lot of information available.

Visit a breast specialist regularly. Get a mammogram as needed. Stay aware of your own body and changes that occur. Check your breasts regularly.

Learn new skills, as bread-making in this book. Learn other new skills as well. When you are focused on what you are doing, you can forget your cancer for that time and even your pain. Help replace what you have lost with the ability to make delicious bread. Nutritious bread is good for you and those you love. Cheer up yourself, family and friends with wonderful bread. Bread is not expensive to make or to give away. People love homemade bread.

Remember that you are still you. You are not breast cancer. There are many breast cancer survivors who have gone through this and are now living happy, loving, contributing lives. They are better people because they survived breast cancer. You can do it, too.

When you recover, reach out to other women with breast cancer and help them as you were helped.

My Breast Cancer Journal

December 20, 2002

Today Dr. Mari told me I have breast cancer. I can have a mastectomy or go to radiation five days a week for six to seven weeks. I think I will choose radiation. Possibly my cancer occurred because I took estrogen for so many years. I am grateful our daughters and many others will not take estrogen.

December 21, 2002

Yesterday I felt brave and today I feel sad. I wish my husband would cancel a trip to Central America that we had planned months ago, before realizing I have cancer. The date we planned to go is right after I will finish radiation. I'll talk to him. He'll be sad to miss our trip. The cancer, since detected early, did not spread out of the duct.

The cancer should not spread to the rest of my body, but I am not afraid to die. I know I will go home to God and to many loved ones that I have never met, I hope I can still live a very long life of service. It is nice to journal and perhaps my journal will help others.

December 22, 2002

It is a blessing to have our second to the youngest daughter home. She just graduated from college in Utah. Now she will go to graduate school in Hawaii and live with us. Yesterday I told all our children that I have breast cancer. Everyone seemed OK with it. I was very tired of telling the story so many times, but it had to be done. Today was the first day since Dr. Mari told me about the cancer that I could actually forget about it and life felt quite ordinary, almost anyway! Thanks dear God for many kind blessings. Thanks for letting me have peace again and get a little removed from what is scary. All will be well.

December 26, 2002

I haven't written in a few days. I was very busy with Christmas. I want back to see Dr. Mari. She is so dear. She said the radiation might burn my breast and so to wait until April to see her again. My husband is stressed that I have cancer. I want to help him to relax and be happy. Everyone deals with challenges in different ways. Everyone does the best they can.

December 27, 2002

Such a remarkable thing happened yesterday. I called a lady from the Mindfulness Community to talk to her about mindfulness. I just happened to mention that I was going to have radiation therapy. I did not know that her sister is a holistic nurse in Germany. Her mother and sister both had breast cancer. She suggested that a mastectomy would be easier on my body. She said radiation therapy could be destructive to other parts of my body.

We hung up and I stood by the phone with a prayer in my heart. The phone rang again. A dear friend, who is a nurse and has had extensive experience with breast cancer patients, called to see if I would help her teach a Healing Touch class. She had no idea that I have breast cancer. I asked her opinion about radiation, verses a mastectomy. She said she would advise me to have a mastectomy. She told me it is would be easier on the rest of the body. It was a miracle she called at that moment.

I called to tell my husband that I had decided to get a mastectomy. Now we can still go on our trip to Central America. That made him very happy.

I called Dr. Mari's office to say I would like to have a mastectomy. I didn't get to talk with Dr. Mari, but I think it will be fine, as it was one of the two options she offered me. My surgery will be done on January 6, 2003. I think to change treatment plans has stirred up my insides a little. As I read more about breast cancer, that has, too, but it is OK. I know my life is in God's hands.

I realize the difficulty cancer patients have in choosing their treatment because there are many choices and one must make choices.

December 28, 2002

This continues to be a remarkable experience, one not asked for, but filled with blessings.

Our children and grandchildren have been so nice. Some of them came over today and vacuumed, washed the floors and folded the clothes. The boys raked the leaves in the yard.

One daughter told me everyone will fast and pray for me the Sunday before my surgery. Then my husband and our son-in-laws will give me a blessing with holy oil for the sick. She started to cry. People keep coming over to bring us things. They are so kind. Many do not know what to say. When I tell them I am fine, they look happy. I ask them if I can help them also. It is humbling to be on the receiving end of such kindness and happier to be on the giving end of it.

I called my friend at Kapiolani Women's and Children's Hospital, who is one of the volunteer coordinators. I told her I would miss a couple weeks of clowning. I am a volunteer clown to the children there with our two therapy dogs. She told me she has the same cancer I have. Five weeks ago she had surgery and is now doing radiation. It was another amazing phone conversation.

December 29, 2002

Somehow I do not feel like the same person I was several weeks ago. Something has changed. I think I have a greater awareness of both heaven and earth, more focus to listen compassionately to the stories of others, more love for the little ones, the need to be very quiet and greater gratitude for the presence of God.

December 30, 2002

It was nice to go to church and feel almost normal. I love teaching the little ones. I have a lot to do before next Monday.

December 31, 2002

This morning I woke up way too early. It was so cold and I was dreaming about chopping. I think it is scary to get a breast removed, but it is also OK and still feels like what is best to do. It will be good to talk with Dr. Mari today.

January 1, 2003

Happy New Year. It is amazing how quickly the years go by.

It was good to see Dr. Mari yesterday. It made me cry to explain my change of plans from radiation to mastectomy. She said it is a good choice to take off the breast. She said that the radiation could damage my ribs and heart. I am so grateful for her loving, excellent care. Dr. Mari thinks I will be fine to go on our trip near the end of February.

We had fun playing with the kids and grandkids yesterday.

Yesterday I passed a man in a wheelchair with part of his leg removed. The remaining leg was not covered and dangled from the chair. People are very brave.

So many people tell me they are praying for me. I am blessed to be remembered in their prayers. The power of prayer is very real. People have natural compassion for those who are sick and suffering.

There is a nursing strike at the hospital I will go to. God bless the nursing strike to be over soon.

I am trying to get the house and the dogs cleaned up before my surgery.

January 2, 2003

Time marches on. We had fun eating dinner with our children and grandchildren at a happy, bright Italian restaurant.

I think I am scared to get a breast cut off, but I think it will go well and that I will recover quickly.

January 3, 2003

As time draws closer to the surgery, I am wondering how the kids and my husband will run our house without me for a couple of days. They are all so busy with their own lives. With all the yard work, care of the dogs, house cleaning and cooking I do, I cannot easily be replaced. I guess all will go as best as it can. I need to let go of how that will be. I think when I get home I can still help do many things. The lady where the dogs get their hair cut has also had breast cancer. She is a friendly lady and told me her story and the stories of many of her friends. Our lives are the stories that we share with love.

Our daughter-in-law's mom called me today. Her husband died of cancer. They did not realize that he had cancer until it had spread into his lymph system. He is greatly missed. I talked with my Mom and Dad.

There is a lot to do before Monday morning.

I have realized there is a giant network that supports cancer, in particular breast cancer. I think there are many other serious diseases and problems people have where there is not such a compassionate loving network in place.

My life is so busy with our family. It was sad to stop volunteering at Queen's Hospital and now also to stop being a hospice volunteer. I would love to do volunteer work with the homeless downtown, but I don't know when I would have the time. The increasing number of grandchildren and my desire to be available to our children and their children uses most of my time. I am very grateful that I have been able to continue to be a clown with our dogs and the hospital children. This feels like an extension of the grandchildren and my great love for children. I feel surrounded by the love of many people. This is a very humbling feeling and a gift I always want to return. Thank you dear God, dear family and friends, for such love.

I want to read a little more in my cancer books about what will happen Monday, but I don't have very many spare moments. Maybe I will read more after the mastectomy.

January 4, 2003

My dear friend did Healing Touch on me last night. We prayed together. It was so nice to see her again.

January 5, 2003

Today is Sunday. I will teach the children at church. Later my husband and our son-in-laws will give me a blessing with oil blessed for the sick. Then we will have a picnic in the park.

I have had so much to do that there has been little time to think about the surgery tomorrow. When I do think about it, I feel a little scared, but also I feel God's peace in my heart. Perhaps that peace comes because of all the people praying for me.

January 5, 2003

It was a sweet day at church and deeply touching to be blessed by my husband and all our son-in-laws. It was fun to picnic in the park. My Mom and Dad called. Tomorrow brings a new adventure

January 10, 2003

Dear Ones,

I think I must write today's entry of this journal of my cancer experience as a thank you and information letter. I wish I could write to each of you personally by hand to thank you for your love, prayers, fasting, Healing Touch treatments, cards, food, flowers and many other kindnesses, but I know I would never be able to write so many times.

I think I feel a little overwhelmed by so much kindness to me and to our family. I have realized more than ever before that when one person in a family has a problem or disease, every person in the family has it, but in different ways. Caring for everyone's needs is a necessity.

I had my mastectomy four days, ago. They will biopsy the rest of the breast, but Dr. Mari felt like it was OK. Our stay in the hospital was filled with constant company from dear family members and friends. We received great care from traveling nurses, Most came from the Southern states. They are wonderful nurses and were so kind to us. In the day and a half we were there, we made many new and dear friends. The operation was easier than I expected it to be. I have not had much pain, except from the drain that is still in my breast. Perhaps I can get it out today or tomorrow. There is not much drainage.

I am a little more tired today than yesterday, but I am doing well. I can help quite a bit at home. It is so nice to be home with everyone and the dogs. The dogs are very attentive and such a help with their love.

I pray as in the beautiful hymn by Grace Noll Crowell that we may return your love to you and to others.

> "Because I have been given much, I too must give;
> Because of thy great bounty, Lord, each day I live.
> I will divide my gifts from thee With ev'ry brother that I see,
> Who has the need of help from me."

God bless you all.

Kathy and the Summers Family

January 11, 2003

Dr. Mari pulled out my drain tube today. She was surprised she could take it out so soon. My husband was home for a little while and it was nice to talk with him. Our daughters went to their dance classes. I made bread and watered the plants. Life seems a little more normal. I do things and then rest and do things and rest. People bring us so much food and flowers. We have to share a lot of it because we do not want to waste any of it. It is very kind of them to bring food and it is a great help.

The biopsy on the rest of the breast had no more cancer, but it did have hyperplasia tissue, which can turn into cancer. Dr. Mari said we did the best thing to do the mastectomy. My chest and arm hurt a little and feel tightly pulled together.

January 12, 2003

Each day I am doing so much better. I feel that God has worked a miracle in my behalf.

January 13, 2003

Today I feel a little discouraged. The incision is rather painful now. I think it is just healing. I wish I could do so much more than I can to help everyone.

January 14, 2003

I am getting more energy back. The pain level is tolerable, too. I think the nerves are trying to heal. I didn't take Advil last night, because it doesn't really help. My chest and underarm look pretty cut up. It is a real lesson in humility.

January 15, 2003

Today I feel a little sad. I think I need to process this experience more with God and all will be well. I haven't been able to do that much with my husband because he has had to work so much and is tired and stressed. The kids also seem to have moved on to more happy things to think about. I am grateful that they have.

January 16, 2003

It was a good day today. I could do quite a lot of work today. Life goes on.

January 17, 2003

I really am feeling stronger and will go to help our daughter today and go to our grandson's basketball game tonight.

The volunteer office at Kapiolani Hospital sent us the most beautiful flowers I have ever seen.

January 18, 2003

My friend came to do Healing Touch on me. She has devoted her life to God.

I am feeling better and have more energy. I have felt a major shift these last two days. It was nice to drive to our daughter's house and watch our granddaughters yesterday and to know that I could do that. I have almost full use of my arm again also. I have been thinking about writing the new bread book over as a bread book for breast cancer patients and survivors, as well as for others. The two seem to go together well. Making handmade bread, eating handmade bread and sharing handmade bread are very therapeutic.

January 19, 2003

My chest was sore yesterday and last night, I do not know if I am getting an infection. I will go see Dr. Mari later. It is nice to have more energy and to accomplish things each day.

January 20, 2003

My chest is still quite sore, but if I am busy I do not notice it too much. Our kids stayed with us for a few days.

January 23, 2003

Yesterday, a dear lady came from the Reach to Recovery program of the American Cancer Society. She told me her story of feeling she must get a mammogram. She was told the microcalcification that appeared in her mammogram was not the bad kind. She still insisted on getting a biopsy. It was cancer. She had a mastectomy. Since the cancer was in one lymph node, she also had chemotherapy and radiation. One year later, she had a breast implant. She said that operation caused her such pain that she cried for weeks.

Despite all she has gone through, she is such a positive lady who talked about God in almost every sentence. I listened to her story and felt sorrow for her experiences.

She told me to massage the burning pain I feel in my breast area. I never would have thought to do that. It helps. She had that burning type of pain for a year and even still it hurts her sometimes.

She is like an angel. She said she always tries to find the good things, no matter how bad things get. She told her doctor, when she had to have her hysterectomy, that she hoped she would loose at least ten pounds from the surgery. She looks like a Hawaiian princess with angel wings. I know God sent her.

January 25, 2003

I feel quite normal again. I am able to work hard and do not tire as easily. I am surprised how sore the whole breast area is. The whole area burns constantly. I don't notice it very much when I am busy, but when I rest or sleep it is very painful. I think in time it will go away.

January 25, 2003

Dear Anne,

How are you doing? How are you doing as president of Healing Touch International? I hope you have time for peace, rest and joy with your family.

I want to tell you a story. I had breast cancer a few months ago and also had a mastectomy after a biopsy. I did not need further treatment. The cancer was contained in the milk duct and was detected early. I had taken estrogen for eight years following a hysterectomy. I am glad many doctors no longer advise its use.

The part of this story I wanted to share with you is about the amazing love I received from the Healing Touch community and the Healing Touch treatments I have been given.

I have had a lot of pain and not wanted to take pain medication, except an occasional Advil. Every time I have had a Healing Touch treatment, the pain has gone away for an extended a period of time. I know Healing Touch has helped me to heal and recover so quickly. I have been on a research mission, not of my own choosing, to verify that Healing Touch reduces pain and helps in the healing process. I already knew that Anne, but to experience it personally has been profound and has enhanced my commitment to its use where there is pain and illness.

You know that I believe all healing comes from God and that we are but tools in God's hands.

God bless you dear friend.

With love always,

Kathy

January 28, 2003

Yesterday I went to see Dr. Mari again. I have been having intense pain in my breast area. Going backwards instead of forwards. Dr. Mari said it is normal and the nerves are trying to heal. She said it could last for several months or longer. I have a slight infection in the incision. She told me put to Neosporin ointment on it and gave me a week's worth of Amoxicillin to take. I researched breast pain on the Internet and found some ideas that I can try. I always feel the pain now, but I just carry on. I am not interested in taking medicines for the pain.

January 30, 2003

I am too sleepy to write now, but wanted to say that I have become part of a sisterhood of women who have breast cancer. I want to pass on the love and knowledge that has been given to me to others.

February 5, 2003

I am feeling better now. I do not have much pain and my incision is healing and getting flat. Thank you dear God.

March 17, 2003

We got to take our trip to Central America and it was wonderful. It was like a honeymoon with my husband. Many people there are so poor and humble.

Now my dear friend Lily has breast cancer and I want to love her as I have been loved. God bless Lily.

April 25, 2003

The bread book is nearly finished. Lily will soon begin her chemotherapy. I am sorry she has to go through all of this. God bless all who so courageously carry on as they try to heal from cancer. Give them hope and peace and strength. Bless people everywhere who suffer for any reason. May we all reach out to one another.

October 26, 2003

Many months have passed since I have written. My chest still gets sore sometimes and is a little numb, but I am doing well. Lily finished her chemotherapy and radiation. She is doing well, too. It is amazing how time goes by. It is a miracle that people are able to heal.

Now my Dad has cancer and I can help him.

One day there will be better treatments for cancer. They will effect the cancer specifically and not the whole body. There are many who spend their lives working towards this goal. God bless their efforts.

Equipment

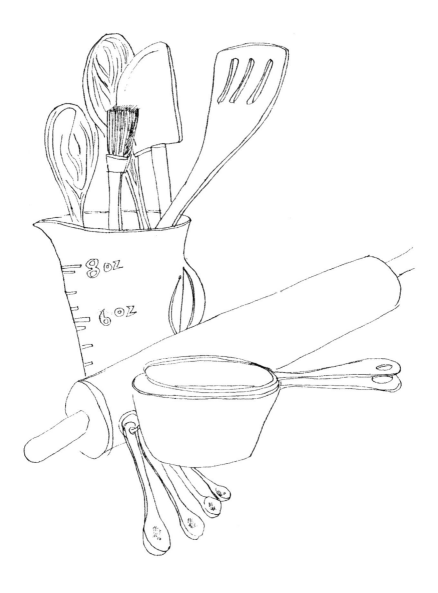

Equipment

Take good care of your equipment. Keep it clean and put away after you have finished using it. Keep your oven, kitchen counters, kitchen cupboards and refrigerator, clean and organized. Taking care of your tools and your kitchen make bread-making an even nicer experience each time you do it.

Useful Equipment to Make Bread

An apron

An easy-to-clean, flat, smooth, work surface at a comfortable height for stirring and kneading. This can be your kitchen counter top or a wooden or plastic cutting board.

A large bowl for mixing the dough

Two medium bowls for making muffins

Graduated measuring cups for measuring the dry ingredients (1 cup, ½ cup, ⅓ cup, ¼ cup)

A clear plastic or glass measuring cup for measuring the liquid ingredients

Measuring spoons

A fork for sifting through the flour before it is measured

A serving spoon for spooning flour into the measuring cups

A table knife for leveling the dry ingredients

A large sturdy mixing spoon

A balloon whisk for stirring the liquid ingredients for muffins

A spatula to scrape all the ingredients from the sides of the bowl when making muffins

A sharp knife for cutting the dough into pieces

A sharp, serrated bread knife for slashing the dough and cutting the bread. Take good care of this knife. Do not use it for anything else.

A straight edged metal pancake turner to keep the work surface clean and smooth, to lift bread off the baking sheet and to help remove bread from the loaf pans

A rolling pin to roll out the dough for cinnamon bread and cinnamon rolls

A candy or other type of cooking thermometer to test the water temperature to dissolve the yeast

An oven thermometer to check the temperature of the oven

A saucepan for boiling water to place in the oven when making French bread

A spray bottle for spraying the crust with water for French bread

Two 9x5x3-inch loaf pans

A 16½x11x½-inch heavy-duty aluminum baking sheet for French bread, challah bread, rolls, pretzels, pizza and focaccia. Use a smaller baking sheet if necessary to fit your oven size.

Baking parchment to put the dough on while baking, instead of using grease. This paper is especially nice to use on the large flat baking sheet. It can be used several times. Baking parchment can be used in any pan, including the loaf pans.

A 13x9x2-inch pan to make pan rolls

A 2½-inch standard-size muffin tin and 3¼-inch muffin tin for large muffins

An 8x8-inch pan for gingerbread and oat cakes

A pastry brush for glazing the bread or rolls

A tape measure or ruler to measure the size of the rolled-out dough

A timer to check the bread's cooking progress at various suggested times

Potholders

A wire cooling rack

A cutting board for slicing the bread

Plastic wrap to loosely cover the rising bread or rolls and to wrap the bread in before freezing it

Plastic zip-lock bags for storing the bread

Paper bags for storing French bread

Heavy-duty freezer zip-lock bags for freezing the bread

INGREDIENTS

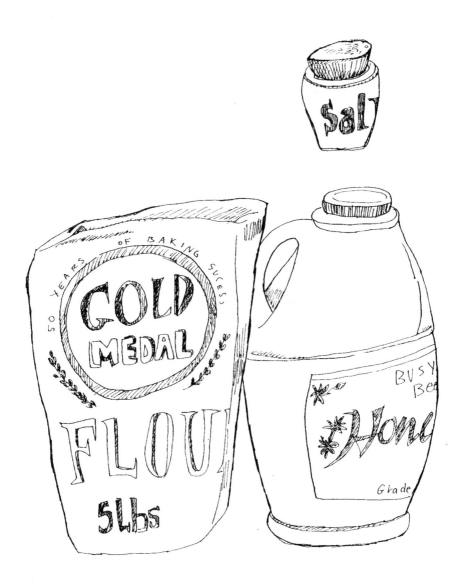

Ingredients

Most of the ingredients can be purchased from a regular grocery store, but some of the ingredients you will find only at a health food grocery store. Health food grocery stores are now a booming business and are delightful places to shop.

Leaven

Leaven is the substance that makes the dough or batter rise.

Yeast, a tiny fungus, is activated by warm water between 110 to 115 degrees. The yeast starts multiplying rapidly. The yeast is fed by the sweetener. The bi-product of this activity is carbon dioxide bubbles that get trapped in the stretchy gluten structure of the wheat based bread dough. This is what makes the bread rise.

I use instant yeast in all the yeast recipes. I use saf-instant yeast made by Lesaffre. It can be purchased at a kitchen store. This yeast rises much faster than regular yeast. It is packaged in a freeze-dried container that weighs a little more than 1 pound. The package is hard and airtight, until you open it, at which point it turns into granules. Once opened, it must be kept in an airtight container in the refrigerator. The yeast will stay active for 3 months. Unopened yeast can be kept frozen in the freezer for 6 months.

Fleischmann's makes an instant yeast called Fleischmann's RapidRise Yeast. Red Star makes instant yeast called RED STAR QUICK-RISE Yeast. These can be purchased at a grocery store. One packet of yeast contains one tablespoon of yeast. The yeast is more expensive when you buy it in the packets rather than in the freeze-dried, larger package.

Baking powder makes the muffin batter rise. It is activated by the liquid ingredients and gives off carbon dioxide bubbles. It reacts when mixed with liquid and then a second time when it is heated in the oven.

Baking soda is used in the gingerbread and oat cake recipes to make the batters rise as it gives off carbon dioxide bubbles.

Liquids

Warm liquid is needed to dissolve and activate the yeast.

Bread made with **water** has a crisp crust, a coarse chewy texture and a pure flavor.

Bread made with **milk** has a velvety grain and an inviting brown crust.

Bread made with **buttermilk** has a fine texture. Buttermilk is skim milk that has bacteria cultures added to thicken it and to give it a sour taste.

Juice adds flavor and sweetness.

Tomato sauce is used as a pizza sauce.

Wheat Flour

Wheat flour, which contains gluten, is the fundamental ingredient in any yeast bread. Gluten is the part of the wheat kernel, which stretches around the carbon dioxide bubbles produced by the yeast. Whole-wheat flour, bread flour and unbleached all-purpose flour are all considered wheat flour.

The amount of flour needed will vary depending on the humidity of the day, the moisture in the flour itself and the way the flour was milled.

Store all flour in a cool place in airtight containers. Whole grain flour should be refrigerated, if possible. Flour can be stored in the refrigerator in airtight containers for 3 months and in the freezer for 6 months. If you bake frequently, it is good to store extra bread flour and whole-wheat flour because you will use them the most.

Almost every large grocery store now sells bread flour and whole-wheat flour. Often you can choose between stone-ground and regularly milled flour. Stone ground flour has a coarser texture.

Whole-wheat flour is ground from the entire wheat kernel: the endosperm, the germ and the bran. It has many nutrients and is heavier and more perishable than bread flour or unbleached all-purpose flour.

Wheat germ is high in fiber and nutrition. Wheat germ is removed from flour that is white in color. Because of its fat content, it must be stored in the refrigerator.

Wheat bran is the outer shell of the wheat kernel. It is a good source of fiber.

Bread flour is white flour with a high amount of gluten in it. This flour is made from the endosperm of the wheat kernel. The gluten increases the elasticity of the dough and results in loaves with higher volume than bread baked with unbleached all-purpose flour.

Unbleached all-purpose flour can be used interchangeably with bread flour. This flour is best to use for muffins. Unbleached all-purpose flour has been refined, but has no added chemicals or preservatives.

Semolina flour is used to make pasta. It is high in protein and is a wonderful addition to French bread.

Other Grain Flour, Flakes and Cereal

Rye flour has a strong flavor and contains some gluten.

Oat flour adds softness and a sweet flavor to bread.

Oatmeal adds a moist, chewy texture. Oats are high in protein and minerals.

Eight-grain cereal or any kind of multi-grain cereal adds texture and nutrition.

Non-grain Flour and Flakes

Cornmeal is ground from yellow or white corn.

Soy flour, ground from whole soybeans, adds important protein and fiber.

Buckwheat flour has a strong flavor. It is a good source of calcium.

Flaxseed meal adds fiber and nutrition.

Mashed potato flakes make the bread softer.

Salt

Use 1 teaspoon salt to every 3 to 4 cups of flour. The amount of salt can vary depending on your taste or health needs. Salt controls the growing yeast. Salt enhances the flavor of the bread. I use **iodized salt**.

Rock salt has larger particles than regular salt.

Sweetener

Sweetener provides food for the yeast to grow and also gives flavor and color to the bread. Vary the amount of sweetener to suit your taste or health needs.

Honey is a sweet golden-brown fluid produced by bees from the nectar of flowers.

Maple syrup is syrup made from the sap of the sugar maple. It has a wonderful flavor in bread and can be used interchangeably with honey.

Brown sugar, which contains molasses, is moist and firm.

Granulated sugar is a refined sugar that has all the molasses removed from it.

Molasses is removed from sugar during the refining process. It has a strong, sweet taste.

Powdered sugar is finely ground sugar that has cornstarch added to it to make it easier to blend. It is used in the glaze for cinnamon rolls.

Malt and malt syrup are made from barley and are excellent sweeteners.

Fat

Fat makes the bread tender, moist and flavorful.

I use **light olive oil** in almost all my baking. Other oils can be used as **canola oil**.

Butter adds wonderful flavor.

Solid white vegetable shortening is used to grease the pans.

Eggs

Eggs add tenderness, richness, flavor, color and protein to the bread.

Spices

allspice
cinnamon
garlic salt
ginger
Italian
pumpkin pie spice

Extracts

almond
vanilla

Nuts

Nuts are a source of protein and high in fat.
almonds
macadamia nuts
pecans

Seeds

caraway
fennel
flax
whole raw millet
poppy
sesame
sunflower

Cheese

cheddar
cream

feta
mozzarella
Parmesan

Fresh Fruit

apple
banana
blueberries-fresh or frozen

Fresh Vegetables

broccoli
carrots
garlic
peppers-green and red
onions-red and yellow

Canned Fruit and Vegetables

applesauce
olives
pumpkin
sun dried tomatoes in oil

Dried Fruit

chopped apricots
chopped dates
raisins

TECHNIQUES

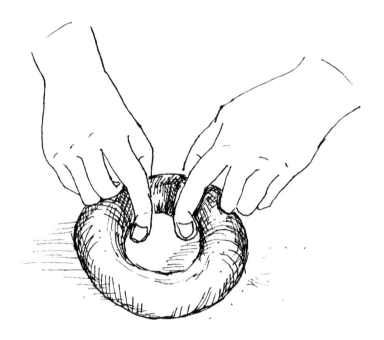

Techniques

Stay Focused

As you stay focused on making the bread, your mind will quiet. Enjoy the peacefulness.

Never Give Up

Remember every new skill takes practice. Don't give up. You'll catch on. We all make mistakes as we learn. Practice will make you an excellent bread-maker. Even the best and most experienced bread-makers fail sometimes.

Read the Recipe

Read the entire recipe before you begin making it. Make sure you have all the ingredients, the equipment and the time to make it. Review the Techniques section if you feel unsure of how to follow the recipe.

Quantity

All the recipes can be doubled, but it is easier to work with smaller amounts of dough.

Prepare the Work Space

Prepare a clean, smooth place, at a comfortable height. You can use a kitchen counter or large wooden or plastic cutting board.

Proof the Yeast

If you are unsure whether the yeast is still active, add 1 teaspoon brown sugar to the yeast mixture. Stir. Allow the mixture to sit for 10 minutes. If the yeast starts to bubble, you can use it. If it doesn't bubble, get new yeast before proceeding further.

Clean as You Work

I like to put away the ingredients as I use them. When I am done with the large mixing bowl, I put soapy water in it and leave it in the sink and put other tools I use inside it. Cleaning up as you work helps the final cleanup to go faster.

Grease

Grease pans with solid white vegetable shortening, Grease the bottom corners and the bottom of the loaf pans especially well. You can sprinkle 1 tablespoon of cornmeal or flour on the bottom of the loaf pan and shake it around. Discard what does not adhere. The thin layer of cornmeal or flour will help the loaf come out more easily. You can slide a metal pancake turner down the sides of the loaf pan to help remove the bread. You can line the loaf pan with baking parchment instead of greasing it.

I love using baking parchment for the bread and rolls made on the flat baking sheet. I prefer this to greasing. Baking parchment can be used in any of the pans, including the loaf pans.

Measure the Ingredients

I have taught hundreds of people how to bake bread. The only two people who were not successful were two ladies who both refused to measure carefully. When you are a beginner, you need to measure carefully.

All ingredients should be measured level.

In case too much salt comes out, as it often does, do not measure the salt over the mixing bowl.

Use full cups of the liquid ingredients. Check the amount at eye level.

Measure the Flour

Adding just the right amount of flour is the hardest thing to learn in making bread.

Sift through the flour several times with a fork, before measuring it. If the flour is packed together you will get too much flour in each cup.

Use a serving spoon to scoop the flour into the measuring cup, until it is overflowing. This takes about 3 to 4 spoonfuls to do. Then with the straight side of a knife, remove the excess flour so that the flour is level with the top of the cup. Measure any type of flour used in this same way.

Mix

Add all the other liquid ingredients (and the sweetener if it is not in liquid form) to the yeast mixture. Stir until well blended. Then add the first amount of flour as directed in the recipe and the salt. Stir until the mixture is thick and smooth.

Gradually add the next amount of flour as you stir. The dough will stick together and pull away from the sides and bottom of the bowl. If the dough does not pull away from the sides and bottom of the bowl, add a little more flour until it does. The dough forms a lump.

Dust

Measure 1 more cup bread flour. Only use what is necessary to knead and shape the dough. Lightly dust the work surface with flour. Place the dough on the work surface.

As you knead, continue to lightly dust the work surface and the dough with flour, so the dough does not get sticky.

Preheat and Check Oven Accuracy

The oven needs to preheat for 20 minutes. When you turn the oven on to preheat it, place the oven thermometer in the middle of the middle rack of the oven. After 20 minutes, read the oven thermometer. You may need to adjust the temperature. Many ovens do not bake at the temperature the dial indicates. This only needs to be done occasionally.

Knead

To knead the dough, fold it over in half towards you and push it down and away from you with the heels of your hands. Use your arms and body to push it down. Turn the dough one-quarter turn. Repeat this fold, push and turn process for about 5 minutes. Sometimes I place one hand over the other to push the dough down. You will develop your own style and rhythm of kneading. Knead until the dough is smooth and elastic.

If dry clumps of flour stick to your hands, wash and dry your hands. Your hands and the work surface should be smooth to knead and to shape the dough. If the work surface gets clumps of dough stuck to it, scrape them off with the flat end of a metal pancake turner and throw them away.

Too Busy to Shape the Dough Now

The dough for any of these recipes can be made through the kneading step and then placed in an oiled bowl. Cover the top of the bowl with plastic wrap or tin foil and put it in the refrigerator for several hours or overnight. Then start the process from the shaping step. Sometimes I don't have time to shape, rise and bake the bread immediately, but it helps to have it already mixed and kneaded. Keep in mind that because the dough is cold, it will take longer to rise.

Shape

I encourage you to make your bread look lovely. Take the time to shape the loaves or rolls nicely. Beautiful bread that tastes good is a work of art.

Bread Baked in Loaf Pans

Cut the dough into 2 equal pieces. Shape each piece into a ball with the smoothest part as the outside of the ball. Tuck the dough under to form the ball. Do not tear the outside surface of the dough as you tuck it under. Let the 2 balls rest on the counter for 5 minutes, so they will be easier to work with as you form the loaves.

Keep the work surface and the dough lightly floured. Place the smooth side of the ball face down on the work surface. Next press the air out of the dough with your hands and form it into a rectangle, approximately 9x5-inches. Starting with the 5-inch side nearest you, firmly, but without tearing the outer surface of the dough, roll the dough away from you into a log. Pinch the seam together and push it into the loaf. Push in and tuck under the two ends of the loaf. Place the dough in the loaf pan, seam side down. Adjust the shape so the loaf is uniform. Repeat with the second ball.

Free Standing Loaves
See French bread recipe.

Braided Loaves
See challah bread recipe.

Round Rolls
Cut the dough into the number of pieces suggested in the recipe and let them rest on the work surface for a couple of minutes. To make a round roll, make a ball, using the smoothest part of the dough as the outside of the ball. Without tearing the outside of the dough, tuck the dough under to form the ball. Place on the baking sheet.

Pan Rolls
Pan rolls are made by forming the dough into balls and placing them close to one another in a 9x13x2-inch pan. The rolls will touch one another as they rise and as they bake. Makes 12 large rolls. Place the rolls 3 across and 4 down. Once they have cooked and cooled, pull them apart.

Knots
Cut the dough into the number of pieces suggested in the recipe and roll each into a 9-inch rope. Tie the rope into a loose knot.

Crescent Rolls
Crescent rolls are made by forming 2 large balls with the dough and allowing them to sit for 2 to 3 minutes. Use the smoothest part of the ball for the outside of the circle. Using your hands and a rolling pin, on a lightly floured surface, roll the ball out to a circle with a 12-inch diameter. Brush the flattened circle with 1 tablespoon of melted butter. As like you would cut a pie, cut the dough into 8 to 12 wedges. Starting at the wide side of the wedge, roll the dough up to the point. Place the junction of the point on the roll, downside on the pan. Repeat with the other ball.

Pretzels
See pretzel recipe and diagram.

Rise

All recipes in this book are designed to save you time by using instant yeast. The instant yeast raises the dough in half the time of regular yeast. The recipes skip the first rising of the dough before shaping it. The dough is shaped and then allowed to rise.

Note carefully the size of the dough after you have shaped it. For bread, let the dough rise until almost double in size. For rolls, let the dough rise until double in size. Usually rising takes about 10 to 15 minutes, but the time can vary. The dough will rise even further while baking, a process called oven spring. It is important not to let the dough rise too high before putting it in the oven or it will fall in the oven, instead of rising more.

Rising depends on the temperature of your kitchen, how much yeast you have used and the ingredients in the dough. Whole grain bread dough rises more slowly than bread dough that uses only bread flour. Dough with oil, eggs, milk, fruit or nuts takes longer to rise than dough that does not contain these ingredients.

If the kitchen is very cool, you can turn the oven on to 400 degrees for 1 minute. Then turn it off and place the pan or pans on the center rack of the oven. Close the oven door and let the dough rise. Remove the dough when it has begun to rise, so you can preheat the oven for baking it.

To help the dough rise faster, you can also place it in an unheated oven with a pan of hot water underneath it.

Glaze

The crust of any bread can be cooked as is or can be enhanced in several different ways:

The crust can be gently brushed with an egg beaten with 1 tablespoon water. This glaze is the best for keeping seeds, minced vegetables, etc., stuck to the crust. It will also give the crust a nice golden shine.

The crust can be gently brushed with an egg white beaten with 1 tablespoon water.

Brushing the crust with butter or olive oil will make a shiny, soft crust.

Spray the crust with water and then very lightly sprinkle the crust with rock salt. Spraying the bread with water every 10 minutes during the baking time, will result in a hard, chewy crust.

Toppings

Top the bread with seeds, minced garlic or onions, rock salt, feta cheese, Parmesan cheese, grated cheese, etc. See recipes for further details.

Bake

Bread should bake on only one oven shelf at a time. Bread loaves and rolls should be placed in the middle of the oven on the middle rack. Pizza and focaccia should be placed on the lowest rack of the oven. Leave space between pans and all the way around pans to allow the heat to circulate.

Do not open the oven during the first 10 minutes of baking because the dough is completing the rising process. After it is complete, you may briefly open the oven door to check the browning of the bread. Some ovens are warmer in the back, front or on one side. Halfway through the baking time. rotate the pan or pans. Turn what is in the front to the back. Change the side the pans are on. Check the bread and rolls 5 minutes before the suggested minimal baking time.

When finished, loaf bread should be nicely browned on the top, sides and bottom and have begun to pull away from the sides of the pan. The bread should sound hollow when you tap the top and the bottom with your finger. Rolls should be golden brown on the tops and the bottoms.

Cool

Remove the bread from the pans or pan immediately. Cool on a wire cooling rack. There must be air space around the entire loaf or loaves, including the bottoms, so they do not get soggy as they cool. Cool for 20 minutes before cutting. As the bread cools, it is actually still cooking and completing the baking process.

Place the rolls on the wire cooling rack, so the bottoms of the rolls do not get wet. Rolls are very good eaten warm.

Muffins need to be cooled in their muffin tins for 5 minutes on a wire cooling rack. Berry muffins should be cooled in the muffin tins for 10 minutes. Then remove the muffins from the muffin tins and place them on a wire cooling rack. Eat warm or further cool.

Write Notes

Write notes on the recipe pages: the amount of bread flour you used, the rising time, the baking temperature, the baking time and any changes to the recipe. If you do not write notes, you may forget. These factors may still vary from time to time. If things did not go well, read the section; Things That Can Go Wrong and How to Fix Them.

Slice

When the bread is cool, slice it on a breadboard with a serrated knife, using a sawing motion, so you do not squash the bread.

Thank

Give thanks for the bread. A grateful heart makes the bread so much better.

Share

Share the bread with others. There is nothing that tastes quite so full of love as homemade bread. Some of the best bread in the world is made with simple and inexpensive ingredients. Bread is always a wonderful gift to give away.

Store

Bread must be completely cool before storing it.

French bread should be stored in a paper bag rather than a plastic bag. It should be frozen or eaten by the second day.

Bread that contains oil or eggs or milk stays fresh longer. It can be stored in a cool place in a plastic bag for 2 days.

Freeze

Bread that you are not going to eat in the first 2 days should be kept in the freezer. The bread must be completely cooled before freezing it. Consider slicing the bread before freezing it, so you can take out individual slices, rather than a whole loaf. Wrap the bread, rolls, pretzels, muffins, etc. tightly in plastic wrap and then place them in heavy plastic freezer zip-lock bag. Try to get the air out of the bag before closing it. Write the date on the bag with a permanent marker. Bread can be kept in the freezer for 3 months.

Defrost

Defrost the bread by taking it out of the zip-lock bag and plastic wrap. Shake off any ice crystals. You can defrost the bread at room temperature on a kitchen towel or wrap a piece of bread in a paper towel and place it in a microwave oven for 15 seconds. Sliced bread can also be toasted to defrost it. An individual roll, pretzel or muffin can be wrapped in a paper towel and placed in a microwave oven for 20 to 30 seconds.

Practice

In a couple of days, try making the same bread again. Practice will teach you to make excellent bread.

How to Use the Recipes

I suggest making the first recipe in each section, before going on to the others. Then try making the variations and the other recipes in each section. With practice, you will learn many of the steps by memory and by feel.

Invent Your Own Recipes

As you become more experienced, be creative. Bread-making is a very flexible art. You can use a different liquid, vary the amount of sweetener, use a different sweetener or not use a sweetener. You can add less salt or omit the salt. You can change the fat, try different flour and combinations of flour. You can add extra ingredients to the recipe, such as cheese, vegetables, dried fruits, nuts, spices, seasonings, herbs, etc. You can experiment with various glazes.

You can use any combinations of flour you like, but at least half of the flour in any yeast bread must be bread flour, unbleached all-purpose flour or whole-wheat flour. Bread flour and unbleached all-purpose flour can be used interchangeably. You can add rye flour, rice flour, soy flour, cornmeal, raw oatmeal, oat flour, oat bran, wheat germ, mashed potato flakes, cooked cereal, etc., to any recipe.

Make bread to suit your taste and heath needs. Have fun!

Use Other Recipes and Make Them This Simple Way

You can take almost any recipe you find, except for sour dough bread, and make it in this same easy way.

1. Dissolve the instant yeast in warm water.

2. Add the sweetener and all the liquid ingredients to the yeast mixture. Allow any hot ingredients to cool first, before adding them to the yeast mixture. Slightly warm any cold ingredients, before adding them to the yeast mixture. Stir.

3. Add about ⅓ of the flour and the salt. Stir until the mixture is thick and smooth.

4. Add enough flour, so the dough forms a lump and leaves the sides and bottom of the bowl.

5. Measure 1 more cup of flour. You will only use a small amount of this flour for dusting as you knead and shape the dough. Knead the dough for 5 minutes.

6. Shape the dough.

7. Let the dough rise. There is no first rising of the dough before shaping it.

8. Bake the dough.

9. Let the bread cool.

10. Slice if necessary.

11. Give thanks. Eat some. Share some.

Things That Can Go Wrong and How to Fix Them

The dough did not rise.

The yeast may no longer be active. Test your yeast. If it does not bubble, get new yeast.

Was the water too hot that you dissolved the yeast in? Water should be between 110 to 115 degrees. If the water is too hot, it kills the yeast.

Be sure that at least half of the flour used was some form of wheat flour.

The bread fell instead of rose in the oven.

The dough may have risen too high before you put it in the oven.

The free form bread did not hold its shape and is rather flat.

The dough was too soft to hold its shape. It needed more flour.

The bread baked unevenly.

Turn the bread once during baking. Put the part of the pan that was in the back in the front. Change the side of the oven the pans are on if there is more than one pan.

The crust is too pale.

The oven temperature was not high enough.

The bread did not bake long enough.

The crust is too dark.

The bread baked too long.

The oven temperature was too high.

Be sure you are baking the bread on middle shelf in the middle of the oven.

The bread is too heavy.

Use less flour.

Use less whole-wheat flour and more bread flour.

The center of the bread is still raw.

The bread needed to cook longer.

Try cooking the bread 25 degrees higher next time.

The dough is too dry.

Bake for less time.

The bread has lines of flour in it.

The dough was not kneaded thoroughly.

The flavor isn't good.

Did you forget to add the salt?

The bread is too salty.

Add less salt.

The bread is too sweet.

Add less sweetener.

RECIPES

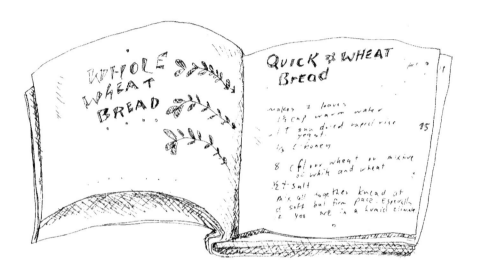

Whole Grain Bread

All the recipes in this section can also be made as rolls.

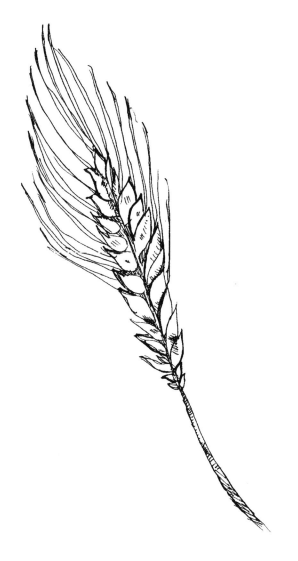

Whole-wheat Bread

An excellent bread for sandwiches and toast.

Yield

two 9x5-inch loaves
or
12 large or 16 medium rolls

Ingredients

2¼ cups warm water
2 tablespoons instant yeast
⅓ cup honey
⅓ cup light olive oil
3 cups whole-wheat flour
2 teaspoons salt
2 to 3 cups bread flour

As you stay focused on making the bread, your mind will quiet. Enjoy the peacefulness.

Instructions

1. First read the recipe. If you need more help, read the Techniques section.

2. Grease two 9x5-inch loaf pans with solid white vegetable shortening. For rolls, cover the baking sheet with a piece of baking parchment or grease the baking sheet.

3. Pour 2¼ cups warm water into a large mixing bowl. Sprinkle 2 tablespoons yeast over the water. Stir until the yeast dissolves.

4. Add ⅓ cup honey and ⅓ cup light olive oil to the yeast mixture. Stir until well blended.

5. In the flour bin, before measuring the flour, sift through the flour several times with a fork.

Use a serving spoon to scoop the flour into the measuring cup, until it is overflowing. Then with the straight side of a knife, remove the excess flour so that the flour is level with the top of the cup. Measure any type of flour this way.

6. Add 3 cups whole-wheat flour and 2 teaspoons salt to the yeast mixture. Stir until the mixture is thick and smooth.

7. Gradually add 2 cups bread flour, stirring with a spoon. The dough will stick together and pull away from the sides and bottom of the bowl. If the dough does not pull away from the sides and bottom of the bowl, add a little more flour until it does. The dough forms a lump.

8. Preheat the oven to 350 degrees.

9. Measure 1 more cup bread flour. Only use what is necessary to knead and shape the dough. Lightly dust the work surface with flour. Place the dough on the work surface. Lightly dust the dough with flour and begin to knead.

10. As you knead, continue to lightly dust the work surface and the dough with flour, so the dough does not get sticky. Knead the dough for about 5 minutes, until it is smooth and elastic.

11. If you are making loaves, cut the dough into 2 equal pieces. Shape each piece into a ball. Let the 2 balls rest on the work surface for 5 minutes before forming the loaves. If you are making rolls, cut the dough into 12 to 16 pieces. Let the pieces rest on the work surface for 5 minutes before shaping further.

12. Keep the work surface and the dough lightly floured. Shape the dough into 2 loaves or 12 to 16 rolls. If you need help with how to shape the loaves or rolls, see Shape in the Techniques section. Place the dough in the loaf pans, seam side down, or place the rolls on the baking sheet.

13. Let the loaves rise until almost double in size. Let the rolls rise until double in size. Usually this takes about 10 to 15 minutes. Place the loaves or rolls into the oven.

14. Bake the loaves for 30 to 40 minutes or until nicely browned on the top, sides and bottom. Bake the rolls for 18 to 22 minutes or until golden brown

on the tops and bottoms. Check the loaves or rolls halfway through the baking time. Rotate the pans or pan in the middle of the baking time for more even baking.

15. When the loaves have finished baking, immediately take them out of the pans and cool them on a wire cooling rack. The loaves need to cool for 20 minutes before slicing them. If you are making rolls, use a pancake turner to take the rolls off the baking sheet and place them on the cooling rack. Rolls can be eaten warm.

16. When the bread is cool, slice it on a breadboard with a serrated knife. Use a sawing motion as you cut, so you do not squash the bread.

17. Give thanks. Eat some. Share some.

18. Write notes on the recipe about the amount of bread flour you used, the rising time, the baking temperature, the baking time and any changes you made to the recipe. If things did not go well, read the section; Things That Can Go Wrong and How to Fix Them.

19. In a couple of days, make this recipe again. Practice will teach you to make excellent bread.

Variations

Follow all the steps for whole-wheat bread, except where new directions are given.

Milk/Wheat Bread

3. Pour 1¼ cups warm water into a large mixing bowl. Sprinkle 2 tablespoons yeast over the water. Stir until the yeast dissolves. Add 1 cup slightly warm milk. Stir.

Buttermilk/Wheat Bread

3. Pour 1¼ cups warm water into a large mixing bowl. Sprinkle 2 tablespoons yeast over the water. Stir until the yeast dissolves. Add 1 cup slightly warm buttermilk. Stir.

Whole-wheat/Nut Bread

6. Add 3 cups whole-wheat flour, 2 teaspoons salt and ¾ cup chopped macadamia nuts or ¾ cup chopped pecans to the yeast mixture. Stir until the mixture is thick and smooth.

Whole-wheat/Sunflower Seed Bread

6. Add 3 cups whole-wheat flour, 2 teaspoons salt and ¾ cup sunflower seeds to the yeast mixture. Stir until the mixture is thick and smooth.

Wheat Germ Bread

6. Add 1 cup raw wheat germ, 2 cups whole-wheat flour, and 2 teaspoons salt to the yeast mixture. Stir until the mixture is thick and smooth.

Wheat Bran Bread

6. Add 1 cup wheat bran, 2 cups whole-wheat flour, and 2 teaspoons salt to the yeast mixture. Stir until the mixture is thick and smooth.

Cornmeal/Wheat

6. Add 1 cup corn meal, 2 cups whole-wheat flour, and 2 teaspoons salt to the yeast mixture. Stir until the mixture is thick and smooth.

Buckwheat Bread

6. Add 1 cup buckwheat flour, 2 cups whole-wheat flour, and 2 teaspoons salt to the yeast mixture. Stir until the mixture is thick and smooth.

Eight-grain Cereal Bread

6. Add 1 cup eight-grain or any kind of multi-grain cereal, 2 cups whole-wheat flour and 2 teaspoons salt to the yeast mixture. Stir until the mixture is thick and smooth.

Potato/Wheat Bread

6. Add 1 cup instant mashed potato flakes, 2 cups whole-wheat flour and 2 teaspoons salt to the yeast mixture. Stir until the mixture is thick and smooth.

100% Whole-wheat Bread

Delicious! A favorite.

Yield

two 9x5-inch loaves
or
12 large or 16 medium rolls

Ingredients

2¼ cups warm water
2 tablespoons instant yeast
⅓ cup molasses
⅓ cup light olive oil
4¾ cups to 5¾ cups whole-wheat flour
2 teaspoons salt

Instructions

1. Read the recipe.

2. Grease the pans.

3. Pour 2¼ cups warm water into bowl. Sprinkle 2 tablespoons yeast over the water. Stir until the yeast dissolves.

4. Add ⅓ cup molasses and ⅓ cup light olive oil to the yeast mixture. Stir.

5. In the flour bin, before measuring the flour, sift through the flour with a fork. Spoon the flour into the cup and level with the straight side of a knife.

6. Add 2¾ cups whole-wheat flour and 2 teaspoons salt to the yeast mixture. Stir.

7. Gradually add 2 cups whole-wheat flour, stirring with the spoon. The dough will stick together and pull away from the sides and bottom of the bowl. If the dough does not do this, add a little more flour until it does.

8. Preheat the oven to 350 degrees.

9. Measure 1 more cup whole-wheat flour. Only use what is necessary to knead and shape the dough. Lightly dust the work surface with flour. Place the dough on the work surface. Lightly dust the dough with flour and begin to knead.

10. As you knead, continue to lightly dust the work surface and the dough with flour. Knead the dough for about 5 minutes.

11. Cut the dough into 2 equal pieces for bread and shape each piece into a ball. For rolls, cut the dough into 12 to 16 pieces. Let the dough rest for 5 minutes.

12. Keeping the work surface and the dough lightly floured, shape the dough into 2 loaves or rolls. Place the dough in the loaf pans, seam side down, or place the rolls on the baking sheet.

13. Let the loaves rise until almost double in size. Let the rolls rise until double in size. Place the loaves or rolls into the oven.

14. Bake the loaves for 30 to 40 minutes or until nicely browned on the top, sides and bottom. Bake the rolls for 18 to 22 minutes or until golden brown on the tops and bottoms. Check the loaves or rolls halfway through the baking time. Rotate the pans or pan in the middle of the baking time for more even baking.

15. When the loaves have finished baking, take the loaves out of the pans and cool them on a wire cooling rack. When the rolls are finished baking, remove them from the baking sheet to the cooling rack. Rolls can be eaten warm.

16. When the bread is cool, slice it on a breadboard with a serrated knife.

17. Give thanks. Eat some. Share some.

18. Write notes on the recipe, if you make any changes.

Multi-grain Bread

A hearty bread that combines the flavors and textures of multi-grain.

Yield

two 9x5-inch loaves
or
12 large or 16 medium rolls

Ingredients

2¼ cups warm water
2 tablespoons instant yeast
⅓ cup honey
1 tablespoon molasses
⅓ cup light olive oil
¼ cup flaxseed meal
¼ cup wheat germ
¼ cup corn meal
¼ cup soy flour
1 cup whole-wheat flour
3 to 4 cups bread flour
2 teaspoons salt

Instructions

1. Read the recipe.

2. Grease the pans.

3. Pour 2¼ cups warm water into bowl. Sprinkle 2 tablespoons yeast over the water. Stir until the yeast dissolves.

4. Add ⅓ cup honey, 1 tablespoon molasses, and ⅓ cup light olive oil to the yeast mixture. Stir.

5. In the flour bin, before measuring the flour, sift through the flour with a fork. Spoon the flour into the cup and level with the straight side of a knife.

6. Add ¼ cup flaxseed meal, ¼ cup wheat germ, ¼ cup cornmeal, ¼ cup soy flour, 1 cup whole-wheat flour, 1 cup bread flour and 2 teaspoons salt to the yeast mixture. Stir.

7. Gradually add 2 cups bread flour, stirring with the spoon. The dough will stick together and pull away from the sides and bottom of the bowl. If the dough does not pull away from the sides and bottom of the bowl, add a little more flour until it does.

8. Preheat the oven to 350 degrees.

9. Measure 1 more cup bread flour. Only use what is necessary to knead and shape the dough. Lightly dust the work surface with flour. Place the dough on the work surface. Lightly dust the dough with flour and begin to knead.

10. As you knead, continue to lightly dust the work surface and the dough with flour. Knead the dough for about 5 minutes.

11. Cut the dough into 2 equal pieces for bread and shape each piece into a ball. For rolls, cut the dough into 12 to 16 pieces. Let the dough rest for 5 minutes.

12. Keeping the work surface and the dough lightly floured, shape the dough into 2 loaves or rolls. Place the dough in the loaf pans, seam side down, or the rolls on the baking sheet

13. Let the loaves rise until almost double in size. Let the rolls rise until double in size. Place the loaves or rolls into the oven.

14. Bake the loaves for 30 to 40 minutes or until nicely browned on the top, sides and bottom. Bake the rolls for 18 to 22 minutes or until golden brown on the tops and bottoms. Check the loaves or rolls halfway through the baking time. Rotate the pans or pan in the middle of the baking time for more even baking.

15. When the loaves have finished baking, take the loaves out of the pans and cool them on a wire cooling rack. When the rolls are finished baking, remove them from the baking sheet to the cooling rack. Rolls can be eaten warm.

16. When the bread is cool, slice it on a breadboard with a serrated knife.

17. Give thanks. Eat some. Share some.

18. Write notes on the recipe, if you make any changes.

High Protein Multi-grain Bread

Wonderful flavor. Good source of protein and fiber.

Yield

two 9x5-inch loaves
or
12 large or 16 medium rolls

Ingredients

2 cups warm water
2 tablespoons instant yeast
⅓ cup honey
⅓ cup light olive oil
1 egg
½ cup dry milk powder
½ cup wheat germ
½ cup soy flour
1 cup whole-wheat flour
3 to 4 cups bread flour
2 teaspoons salt

Instructions

1. Read the recipe.

2. Grease the pans.

3. Pour 2 cups warm water into a large mixing bowl. Sprinkle 2 tablespoons yeast over the water. Stir until the yeast dissolves.

4. Add ⅓ cup honey, ⅓ cup light olive oil and 1 egg to the yeast mixture. Stir.

5. In the flour bin, before measuring the flour, sift through the flour with a fork. Spoon the flour into the cup and level with the straight side of a knife.

6. Add ½ cup dry milk powder, ½ cup wheat germ, ½ cup soy flour, 1 cup whole-wheat flour, 1 cup bread flour to the yeast mixture and 2 teaspoons salt. Stir.

7. Gradually add 2 cups bread flour, stirring with the spoon. The dough will stick together and pull away from the sides and bottom of the bowl. If the dough does not pull away from the sides and bottom of the bowl, add a little more flour until it does.

8. Preheat the oven to 350 degrees.

9. Measure 1 more cup bread flour. Only use what is necessary to knead and shape the dough. Lightly dust the work surface with flour. Place the dough on the work surface. Lightly dust the dough with flour and begin to knead.

10. As you knead, continue to lightly dust the work surface and the dough with flour. Knead the dough for about 5 minutes.

11. Cut the dough into 2 equal pieces for bread and shape each piece into a ball. For rolls, cut the dough into 12 to 16 pieces. Let the dough rest for 5 minutes.

12. Keeping the work surface and the dough lightly floured, shape the dough into 2 loaves or rolls. Place the dough in the loaf pans, seam side down, or the rolls on the baking sheet

13. Let the loaves rise until almost double in size. Let the rolls rise until double in size. Place the loaves or rolls into the oven.

14. Bake the loaves for 30 to 40 minutes or until nicely browned on the top, sides and bottom. Bake the rolls for 18 to 22 minutes or until golden brown on the tops and bottoms. Check the loaves or rolls halfway through the baking time. Rotate the pans or pan in the middle of the baking time for more even baking.

15. When the loaves have finished baking, take the loaves out of the pans and cool them on a wire cooling rack. When the rolls are finished baking, remove them from the baking sheet to the cooling rack. Rolls can be eaten warm.

16. When the bread is cool, slice it on a breadboard with a serrated knife.

17. Give thanks. Eat some. Share some.

18. Write notes on the recipe, if you make any changes.

Seed Bread

A dense, nutritious bread, filled with fiber.

Yield

two 9x5-inch loaves
or
12 large or 16 medium rolls

Ingredients

2¼ cups warm water
2 tablespoons instant yeast
⅓ cup honey
⅓ cup light olive oil
3 cups whole-wheat flour
2 teaspoons salt
1 tablespoon flaxseeds
1 tablespoon fennel seeds
1 tablespoon sesame seeds
1 tablespoon raw whole millet
½ cup sunflower seeds
2 to 3 cups bread flour

Glaze

1 egg, beaten with 1 tablespoon water
Sprinkle with 1 to 2 tablespoons of poppy seeds.

Instructions

1. Read the recipe.

2. Grease the pans.

3. Pour 2¼ cups warm water into bowl. Sprinkle 2 tablespoons yeast over the water. Stir until the yeast dissolves.

4. Add ⅓ cup honey and ⅓ cup light olive oil to the yeast mixture. Stir.

5. In the flour bin, before measuring the flour, sift through the flour with a fork. Spoon the flour into the cup and level with the straight side of a knife.

6. Add 3 cups whole-wheat flour, 2 teaspoons salt, 1 tablespoon flaxseeds, 1 tablespoon fennel seeds, 1 tablespoon sesame seeds, 1 tablespoon raw whole millet and ½ cup sunflower seeds to the yeast mixture. Stir.

7. Gradually add 2 cups bread flour, stirring with the spoon. The dough will stick together and pull away from the sides and bottom of the bowl. If the dough does not pull away from the sides and bottom of the bowl, add a little more flour until it does.

8. Preheat the oven to 350 degrees.

9. Measure 1 more cup bread flour. Only use what is necessary to knead and shape the dough. Lightly dust the work surface with flour. Place the dough on the work surface. Lightly dust the dough with flour and begin to knead.

10. As you knead, continue to lightly dust the work surface and the dough with flour. Knead the dough for about 5 minutes.

11. Cut the dough into 2 equal pieces for bread and shape each piece into a ball. For rolls, cut the dough into 12 to 16 pieces. Let the dough rest for 5 minutes.

12. Keeping the work surface and the dough lightly floured, shape the dough into 2 loaves or rolls. Place the dough in the loaf pans, seam side down, or the rolls on the baking sheet

13. Let the loaves rise until almost double in size. Let the rolls rise until double in size. Glaze with egg mixture. Sprinkle with 1 to 2 tablespoons of poppy seeds. Place the loaves or rolls into the oven.

14. Bake the loaves for 30 to 40 minutes or until nicely browned on the top, sides and bottom. Bake the rolls for 18 to 22 minutes or until golden brown on the tops and bottoms. Check the loaves or rolls halfway through the baking time. Rotate the pans or pan in the middle of the baking time for more even baking.

15. When the loaves have finished baking, take the loaves out of the pans and cool them on a wire cooling rack. When the rolls are finished baking, remove them from the baking sheet to the cooling rack. Rolls can be eaten warm.

16. When the bread is cool, slice it on a breadboard with a serrated knife.

17. Give thanks. Eat some. Share some.

18. Write notes on the recipe, if you make any changes.

Rye Bread

Enjoy the tangy flavor of rye flour and caraway seeds.

Yield

two 9x5-inch loaves
or
12 large or 16 medium rolls.

Ingredients

2¼ cups warm water
2 tablespoons instant yeast
⅓ cup molasses
⅓ cup light olive oil
3 cups dark rye flour
2 teaspoons salt
1 tablespoon caraway seeds
2 to 3 cups bread flour

Instructions

1. Read the recipe.

2. Grease the pans.

3. Pour 2¼ cups warm water into bowl. Sprinkle 2 tablespoons yeast over the water. Stir until the yeast dissolves.

4. Add ⅓ cup molasses and ⅓ cup light olive oil to the yeast mixture. Stir.

5. In the flour bin, before measuring the flour, sift through the flour with a fork. Spoon the flour into the cup and level with the straight side of a knife.

6. Add 3 cups dark rye flour, 2 teaspoons salt and 1 tablespoon caraway seeds to the yeast mixture. Stir.

7. Gradually add 2 cups bread flour, stirring with the spoon. The dough will stick together and pull away from the sides and bottom of the bowl. If the dough does not pull away from the sides and bottom of the bowl, add a little more flour until it does.

8. Preheat the oven to 350 degrees.

9. Measure 1 more cup bread flour. Only use what is necessary to knead and shape the dough. Lightly dust the work surface with flour. Place the dough on the work surface. Lightly dust the dough with flour and begin to knead.

10. As you knead, continue to lightly dust the work surface and the dough with flour. Knead the dough for about 5 minutes.

11. Cut the dough into 2 equal pieces for bread and shape each piece into a ball. For rolls, cut the dough into 12 to 16 pieces. Let the dough rest for 5 minutes.

12. Keeping the work surface and the dough lightly floured, shape the dough into 2 loaves or rolls. Place the dough in the loaf pans seam side down, or the rolls on the baking sheet

13. Let the loaves rise until almost double in size. Let the rolls rise until double in size. Place the loaves or rolls into the oven.

14. Bake the loaves for 30 to 40 minutes or until nicely browned on the top, sides and bottom. Bake the rolls for 18 to 22 minutes or until golden brown on the tops and bottoms. Check the loaves or rolls halfway through the baking time. Rotate the pans or pan in the middle of the baking time for more even baking.

15. When the loaves have finished baking, take the loaves out of the pans and cool them on a wire cooling rack. When the rolls are finished baking, remove them from the baking sheet to the cooling rack. Rolls can be eaten warm.

16. When the bread is cool, slice it on a breadboard with a serrated knife.

17. Give thanks. Eat some. Share some.

18. Write notes on the recipe, if you make any changes.

Oatmeal Raisin Bread

Always a hit. I love to bake with oatmeal.

Yield

two 9x5-inch loaves
or
12 large or 16 medium rolls

Ingredients

1¼ cup warm water
2 tablespoons instant yeast
1 cup slightly warm milk
⅓ cup honey
⅓ cup light olive oil
1 cup oats
1 cup whole-wheat flour
3 to 4 cups bread flour
2 teaspoons salt
1 teaspoon cinnamon
1 cup raisins (If the raisins are hard and dry, soak them in hot water for 10 minutes. Then drain them well, before adding them to the dough.)

Instructions

1. Read the recipe.

2. Grease the pans.

3. Pour 1¼ cups warm water into a large mixing bowl. Sprinkle 2 tablespoons yeast over the water. Stir until the yeast dissolves. Add 1 cup slightly warm milk. Stir.

4. Add ⅓ cup honey and ⅓ cup light olive oil to the yeast mixture. Stir.

5. In the flour bin, before measuring the flour, sift through the flour with a fork. Spoon the flour into the cup and level with the straight side of a knife.

6. Add 1 cup oats, 1 cup whole-wheat flour, 1 cup bread flour, 2 teaspoons salt, 1 teaspoon cinnamon and 1 cup raisins to the yeast mixture. Stir.

7. Gradually add 2 cups bread flour, stirring with a spoon. The dough will stick together and pull away from the sides and bottom of the bowl. If the dough does not pull away from the sides and bottom of the bowl, add a little more flour until it does.

8. Preheat the oven to 350 degrees.

9. Measure 1 more cup bread flour. Only use what is necessary to knead and shape the dough. Lightly dust the work surface with flour. Place the dough on the work surface. Lightly dust the dough with flour and begin to knead.

10. As you knead, continue to lightly dust the work surface and the dough with flour. Knead the dough for about 5 minutes.

11. Cut the dough into 2 equal pieces for bread and shape each piece into a ball. For rolls, cut the dough into 12 to 16 pieces. Let the dough rest for 5 minutes.

12. Keeping the work surface and the dough lightly floured, shape the dough into 2 loaves or rolls. Place the dough in the loaf pans, seam side down, or the rolls on the baking sheet

13. Let the loaves rise until almost double in size. Let the rolls rise until double in size. Place the loaves or rolls into the oven.

14. Bake the loaves for 30 to 40 minutes or until nicely browned on the top, sides and bottom. Bake the rolls for 18 to 22 minutes or until golden brown on the tops and bottoms. Check the loaves or rolls halfway through the baking time. Rotate the pans or pan in the middle of the baking time for more even baking.

15. When the loaves have finished baking, take the loaves out of the pans and cool them on a wire cooling rack. When the rolls are finished baking, remove them from the baking sheet to the cooling rack. Rolls can be eaten warm.

16. When the bread is cool, slice it on a breadboard with a serrated knife.

17. Give thanks. Eat some. Share some.

18. Write notes on the recipe, if you make any changes.

WHITE BREAD

All the recipes in this section can also be made as rolls.

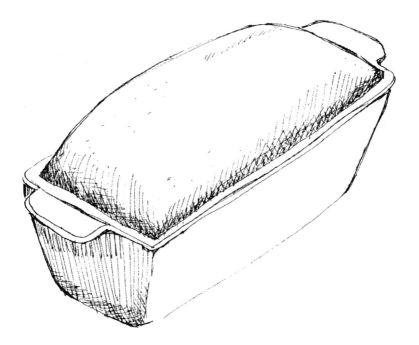

White Bread

Great for sandwiches and toast. Kids love this bread.

Yield

two 9x5-inch loaves
or
12 large or 16 medium rolls

Ingredients

2¼ cups warm water
2 tablespoons instant yeast
¼ cup honey or pure maple syrup
⅓ cup light olive oil
5¼ to 6¼ cups bread flour
2 teaspoons salt

As you stay focused on making the bread, your mind will quiet. Enjoy the peacefulness.

Instructions

1. First read the recipe. If you need more help, read the Techniques section.

2. Grease two 9 by 5-inch loaf pans with solid white vegetable shortening. For rolls, cover the baking sheet with a piece of baking parchment or grease the baking sheet.

3. Pour 2¼ cups warm water into a large mixing bowl. Sprinkle 2 tablespoons yeast over the water. Stir until the yeast dissolves.

4. Add ¼ cup honey and ⅓ cup light olive oil to the yeast mixture. Stir until well blended.

5. In the flour bin, before measuring the flour, sift through the flour several times with a fork.

Use a serving spoon to scoop the flour into the measuring cup, until it is overflowing. Then with the straight side of a knife, remove the excess flour so that the flour is level with the top of the cup. Measure any type of flour this way.

6. Add 3¼ cups bread flour and 2 teaspoons of salt to the yeast mixture. Stir until the mixture is thick and smooth.

7. Gradually add 2 cups bread flour, stirring with a spoon. The dough will stick together and pull away from the sides and bottom of the bowl. If the dough does not pull away from the sides and bottom of the bowl, add a little more flour until it does. The dough forms a lump.

8. Preheat the oven to 350 degrees.

9. Measure 1 more cup bread flour. Only use what is necessary to knead and shape the dough. Lightly dust the work surface with flour. Place the dough on the work surface. Lightly dust the dough with flour and begin to knead.

10. As you knead, continue to lightly dust the work surface and the dough with flour, so the dough does not get sticky. Knead the dough for about 5 minutes, until it is smooth and elastic.

11. If you are making loaves, cut the dough into 2 equal pieces. Shape each piece into a ball. Let the 2 balls rest on the work surface for 5 minutes before forming the loaves. If you are making rolls, cut the dough into 12 to 16 pieces. Let the pieces rest on the work surface for 5 minutes before shaping further.

12. Keep the work surface and the dough lightly floured. Shape the dough into 2 loaves or rolls. If you need help with how to shape the loaves or rolls, see Shape in the Techniques section. Place the dough in the loaf pans, seam side down, or place the rolls on the baking sheet.

13. Let the loaves rise until almost double in size. Let the rolls rise until double in size. Usually this takes about 10 to 15 minutes. Place the loaves or rolls into the oven.

14. Bake the loaves for 30 to 40 minutes or until nicely browned on the top, sides and bottom. Bake the rolls for 18 to 22 minutes or until golden brown

on the tops and bottoms. Check the loaves or rolls halfway through the baking time. Rotate the pans or pan in the middle of the baking time for more even baking.

15. When the loaves have finished baking, immediately take them out of the pans and cool them on a wire cooling rack. The loaves need to cool for 20 minutes before slicing them. If you are making rolls, use a pancake turner to take the rolls off the baking sheet and place on the cooling rack. Rolls can be eaten warm.

16. When the bread is cool, slice it on a breadboard with a serrated knife. Use a sawing motion as you cut, so you do not squash the bread.

17. Give thanks. Eat some. Share some.

18. Write notes on the recipe about the amount of bread flour you used, the rising time, the baking temperature, the baking time and any changes you made to the recipe. If things did not go well, read the section; Things That Can Go Wrong and How to Fix Them.

19. In a couple of days, make this recipe again. Practice will teach you to make excellent bread.

Variations

Follow all the steps for white bread except where new directions are given.

Milk Bread

3. Pour 1¼ cups warm water into a large mixing bowl. Sprinkle 2 tablespoons yeast over the water. Stir until the yeast dissolves. Add 1 cup slightly warm milk. Stir.

Buttermilk Bread

3. Pour 1¼ cups warm water into a large mixing bowl. Sprinkle 2 tablespoons yeast over the water. Stir until the yeast dissolves. Add 1 cup slightly warm buttermilk. Stir.

After removing the loaves or rolls from the oven, brush them with 1 tablespoon melted butter.

Soymilk Bread

3. Pour 1¼ cups warm water into a large mixing bowl. Sprinkle 2 tablespoons yeast over the water. Stir until the yeast dissolves. Add 1 cup slightly warm soymilk. Stir.

Potato Bread

6. Add 1 cup mashed potato flakes, 2¼ cups bread flour and 2 teaspoons of salt to the yeast mixture. Stir until the mixture is thick and smooth.

Cornmeal Bread

6. Add 1 cup cornmeal, 2¼ cups bread flour and 2 teaspoons of salt to the yeast mixture. Stir until the mixture is thick and smooth.

Oatmeal Bread

6. Add 1 cup oatmeal, 2¼ cups bread flour and 2 teaspoons salt to the yeast mixture. Stir until the mixture is thick and smooth.

Wheat Germ Bread

6. Add 1 cup wheat germ, 2¼ cups bread flour and 2 teaspoons salt to the yeast mixture. Stir until the mixture is thick and smooth.

Nutritious White Bread

Excellent nutrition, wonderful taste.

Yield

two 9x5-inch loaves
or
12 large or 16 medium rolls

Ingredients

2 cups warm water
2 tablespoons instant yeast
¼ cup honey
⅓ cup light olive oil
1 egg
½ cup dry milk powder
½ cup wheat germ
½ cup soy flour
4 to 5 cups bread flour
2 teaspoons salt

Instructions

1. Read the recipe.

2. Grease the pans.

3. Pour 2 cups warm water into a large mixing bowl. Sprinkle 2 tablespoons yeast over the water. Stir until the yeast dissolves.

4. Add ¼ cup honey, ⅓ cup light olive oil and 1 egg to the yeast mixture. Stir.

5. In the flour bin, before measuring the flour, sift through the flour with a fork. Spoon the flour into the cup and level with the straight side of a knife.

6. Add ½ cup dry milk powder, ½ cup wheat germ, ½ cup soy flour, 2 cups bread flour and 2 teaspoons of salt to the yeast mixture. Stir.

7. Gradually add 2 cups bread flour, stirring with a spoon. The dough will stick together and pull away from the sides and bottom of the bowl. If the dough does not pull away from the sides and bottom of the bowl, add a little more flour until it does.

8. Preheat the oven to 350 degrees.

9. Measure 1 more cup bread flour. Only use what is necessary to knead and shape the dough. Lightly dust the work surface with flour. Place the dough on the work surface. Lightly dust the dough with flour and begin to knead.

10. As you knead, continue to lightly dust the work surface and the dough with flour. Knead the dough for about 5 minutes.

11. Cut the dough into 2 equal pieces for bread and shape each piece into a ball. For rolls, cut the dough into 12 to 16 pieces. Let the dough rest for 5 minutes.

12. Keeping the work surface and the dough lightly floured, shape the dough into 2 loaves or rolls. Place the dough in the loaf pans, seam side down, or the rolls on the baking sheet

13. Let the loaves rise until almost double in size. Let the rolls rise until double in size. Place the loaves or rolls into the oven.

14. Bake the loaves for 30 to 40 minutes or until nicely browned on the top, sides and bottom. Bake the rolls for 18 to 22 minutes or until golden brown on the tops and bottoms. Check the loaves or rolls halfway through the baking time. Rotate the pans or pan in the middle of the baking time for more even baking.

15. When the loaves have finished baking, take the loaves out of the pans and cool them on a wire cooling rack. When the rolls are finished baking, remove them from the baking sheet to the cooling rack. Rolls can be eaten warm.

16. When the bread is cool, slice it on a breadboard with a serrated knife.

17. Give thanks. Eat some. Share some.

18. Write notes on the recipe, if you make any changes.

French Bread

All the recipes in this section can also be made as rolls.

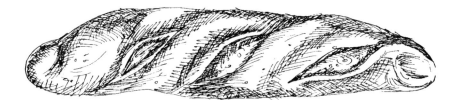

French Bread

People love French bread. It is made with very simple ingredients and is a slightly salty, firm bread with a chewy crust. It makes excellent garlic toast.

Yield

1 long loaf
or
6 large rolls or 8 medium rolls

Ingredients

1½ cups warm water
1 tablespoon instant yeast
1 tablespoon honey
3 to 4 cups bread flour
1½ teaspoons salt
3 to 4 tablespoons of corn meal for sprinkling the baking pan

glaze

a spray bottle with clean water
rock salt
or
1 egg white beaten with 1 tablespoon water

The loaf can be baked on a baking sheet or in a French bread mold. I like using the mold and cover it with baking parchment.

As you stay focused on making the bread, your mind will quiet. Enjoy the peacefulness.

Instructions

1. First read the recipe. If you need more help, read the Techniques section.

2. Cover the baking sheet with a piece of baking parchment or grease the baking sheet with solid white shortening. If you are using a French bread mold, cover it with baking parchment.

3. Pour 1½ cups warm water into a large mixing bowl. Sprinkle 1 tablespoon yeast over the water. Stir until the yeast dissolves.

4. Add 1 tablespoon honey to the yeast mixture. Stir.

5. In the flour bin, before measuring the flour, sift through the flour several times with a fork.

   Use a serving spoon to scoop the flour into the measuring cup, until it is overflowing. Then with the straight side of a knife, remove the excess flour so that the flour is level with the top of the cup. Measure any type of flour this way.

6. Add 2 cups bread flour and 1½ teaspoons of salt to the yeast mixture. Stir until the mixture is thick and smooth.

7. Add 1 cup of bread flour, stirring with the spoon. The dough will stick together and pull away from the sides and bottom of the bowl. If the dough does not pull away from the sides and bottom of the bowl, add a little more flour until it does. The dough forms a lump.

8. Preheat the oven to 400 degrees.

9. Measure 1 more cup bread flour. Only use what is necessary to knead and shape the dough. Lightly dust the work surface with flour. Place the dough on the work surface. Lightly dust the dough with flour and begin to knead.

10. As you knead, continue to lightly dust the work surface and the dough with flour, so the dough does not get sticky. Knead the dough for about 5 minutes, until it is smooth and elastic. When you are finished kneading, the dough should feel firmer than the dough for loaf bread.

11. If you are making a loaf, shape the dough into a ball. Let the ball rest on the work surface for 5 minutes. If you are making rolls, cut the dough into 6 to 8 pieces. Let the pieces rest on the work surface for 5 minutes.

12. Keep the work surface and the dough lightly floured. To form the loaf, place the smoothest side of the ball as the outside surface. With your hands, pat the ball into a rectangle, about 8x12-inches. The exact size does not matter.

Starting with the 12-inch side nearest you, firmly, but without tearing the outer surface of the dough, roll the dough away from you into a log. Pinch the seam together and push into the loaf. Push in and tuck under the two ends of the loaf. Place the loaf seam side down on the baking sheet or mold and adjust the shape so the loaf is uniform. The dough can be divided to make 2 smaller loaves. To make the rolls, use the smoothest part of the dough as the outside of the ball. Tuck the dough under to form a ball. Place the rolls on the baking sheet.

13. Let the loaf rise until almost double in size. Let the rolls rise until double in size. Usually this takes about 10 to 15 minutes.

14. Using a sharp knife, slash the top of the loaf with 4 diagonal slashes, about ¼ inch deep. Slash the rolls with 2 diagonal slashes, about ¼ inch deep.

15. If you are using the water glaze and rock salt, spray the bread with water and lightly sprinkle the top of the bread with rock salt.

    If you are using the egg white glaze, paint the glaze onto the loaf with a pastry brush. Paint the loaf again 5 minutes before it is done.

16. Place a pot of boiling water on the middle shelf of your oven. Place the pan with your loaf of bread or rolls nearby on this same shelf.

17. Bake the loaf for 35 to 40 minutes or until nicely browned on the top, sides and bottom. Bake the rolls for 18 to 22 minutes or until golden brown on the tops and bottoms. Check the loaf or rolls halfway through the baking time. Rotate the pan in the middle of the baking time for more even baking. After rotating the pan, spray the loaf or rolls with water. Continue baking. Spray the loaf or rolls once more 5 minutes before they are done.

18. Immediately remove the loaf from the pan and cool on a wire cooling rack. The loaf needs to cool for 20 minutes before slicing. If you are making rolls, use a pancake turner to take the rolls off the baking sheet and place them on the cooling rack. Rolls can be eaten warm.

19. When the bread is cool, slice it on a breadboard with a serrated knife. Use a sawing motion as you cut, so you do not squash the bread.

20. Give thanks. Eat some. Share some.

21. Write notes on the recipe about the amount of bread flour you used, the rising time, the baking temperature, the baking time and any changes you made to the recipe. If things did not go well, read the section; Things That Can Go Wrong and How to Fix Them.

    French bread should be stored at room temperature in a paper bag, rather than a plastic bag.

    French bread or rolls get stale quickly because there is no oil in the dough. Whatever will not be eaten in the first two days, should be stored in the freezer.

22. In a couple of days, make this recipe again. Practice will teach you to make excellent bread.

Variations

Follow all the steps for French bread except where new directions are given.

Vienna Bread

3. Pour ½ cup of warm water into a large mixing bowl. Add 1 cup slightly warmed milk. Stir. Sprinkle 1 tablespoons yeast over the warm water and milk. Stir until the yeast dissolves.

Semolina French Bread

6. Add 1 cup semolina flour, 1 cup bread flour and 1½ teaspoons salt to the yeast mixture. Stir until the mixture is thick and smooth.

Whole-wheat French Bread

6. Add ¾ cup whole-wheat flour, 1 cup bread flour and 1½ teaspoons salt to the yeast mixture. Stir until the mixture is thick and smooth.

Olive Bread

6. Add ½ cup semolina flour, 1½ cups bread flour, 1 teaspoon salt and ¾ cup sliced black olives. Drain and then pat the olives dry in a paper towel, before adding them to the yeast mixture. Stir until the mixture is thick and smooth.

Cornmeal French Bread

6. Add ½ cup cornmeal, ¼ cup whole-wheat flour, 1 cup bread flour and 1½ teaspoons salt to the yeast mixture. Stir until the mixture is thick and smooth.

Rye French Bread

4. Add 1 tablespoon molasses to the yeast mixture. Stir.

6. Add ¾ cup dark rye flour, 1 cup bread flour, 1½ teaspoons salt and 1 tablespoon of caraway seeds to the yeast mixture. Stir until the mixture is thick and smooth.

Multi-grain/Seed French Bread

4. Add 1 tablespoon honey and 1 tablespoon light olive oil to the yeast mixture. Stir.

6. Add ¾ cup whole-wheat flour, ¼ cup cornmeal, ¼ cup soy flour, ¼ cup wheat germ, ¼ cup rye flour, 1½ teaspoon salt, 1 tablespoon poppy seeds, 1 tablespoon raw whole millet and ¼ cup sunflower seeds to the yeast mixture. Stir until the mixture is thick and smooth.

SWEET BREAD

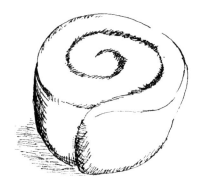

Challah Bread

Challah is a beautiful braided bread of Jewish origin. The eggs, honey and oil make it almost cake-like.

Yield

1 large braided loaf

Ingredients

1 cup warm water
1 tablespoon instant yeast
¼ cup light olive oil
¼ cup brown sugar
2 large eggs
3¼ cups to 4¼ cups flour
1 teaspoon salt

glaze

1 beaten egg

topping

2 tablespoons sesame or poppy seeds for topping

As you stay focused on making the bread, your mind will quiet. Enjoy the peacefulness.

Instructions

1. First read the recipe.

2. Cover the baking sheet with a piece of baking parchment or grease the baking sheet with solid white vegetable shortening.

3. Pour 1 cup warm water into a large mixing bowl. Sprinkle 1 tablespoon yeast over the water. Stir until the yeast dissolves.

4. Add ¼ cup light olive oil, ¼ cup brown sugar and 2 large eggs to the yeast mixture. Stir until well blended.

5. In the flour bin, before measuring the flour, sift through the flour several times with a fork.

   Use a serving spoon to scoop the flour into the measuring cup, until it is overflowing. Then with the straight side of a knife, remove the excess flour so that the flour is level with the top of the cup. Measure any type of flour this way.

6. Add 2¼ cups bread flour and 1 teaspoon salt to the yeast mixture. Stir until the mixture is thick and smooth.

7. Add 1 cup bread flour, stirring with the spoon. The dough will stick together and pull away from the sides and bottom of the bowl. If the dough does not pull away from the sides and bottom of the bowl, add a little more flour until it does. The dough forms a lump.

8. Preheat the oven to 350 degrees.

9. Measure 1 more cup bread flour. Only use what is necessary to knead and shape the dough. Lightly dust the work surface with flour. Place the dough on the work surface. Lightly dust the dough with flour and begin to knead.

10. As you knead, continue to lightly dust the work surface and the dough with flour, so the dough does not get sticky. Knead the dough for about 5 minutes, until it is smooth and elastic.

11. Cut the dough into 3 equal pieces. Shape each piece into a ball by tucking the dough under with the smoothest part as the outside of the ball. Do not tear the outside surface of the dough as you tuck it under. Let the balls rest on the work surface for 5 minutes, so they will be easier to work with as you form the braid.

12. Keep the work surface and the dough lightly floured. Place the smooth side of the ball face down on the work surface. Roll into a 14-inch long rope. Do the same with the other two balls. Next loosely braid the ropes. Pinch each end of the loaf together and tuck under. Place the braid on the baking sheet.

13. Let the loaf rise until almost double in size, a process that usually takes about 10 to 15 minutes.

14. Brush the top of the loaf with a beaten egg and sprinkle it with 2 tablespoons sesame seeds or 2 tablespoons poppy seeds. Place the loaf into the oven.

15. Bake the loaf for 35 to 40 minutes or until golden brown on the top, sides and bottom. Because this is a large loaf, it is important to cook it thoroughly so the center will not be raw. Check the loaf halfway through the baking time. Rotate the pan in the middle of the baking time for more even baking.

16. When the loaf has finished baking, remove the loaf from the baking sheet and cool on a wire cooling rack for 20 minutes before cutting.

17. Give thanks. Eat some. Share some.

18. Write notes on the recipe about the amount of bread flour you used, the rising time, the baking temperature, the baking time and any changes you made to the recipe. If things did not go well, read the section; Things That Can Go Wrong and How to Fix Them.

19. In a couple of days, make this recipe again. Practice will teach you to make excellent bread.

Variations

Follow all the steps for challah bread except where new directions are given.

Whole-wheat Challah Bread

6. Add ¾ cup whole-wheat flour, 1¼ cups bread flour and 1 teaspoon salt to the yeast mixture. Stir until the mixture is thick and smooth.

Cinnamon Bread

Our kids love this cinnamon bread. We use brown sugar instead of white sugar in the cinnamon mixture. People say it is the best cinnamon bread they have ever tasted.

Yield

two 9x5-inch loaves.

Ingredients

1 cup warm water
1 cup slightly warm milk
1 tablespoon instant yeast
¼ cup light olive oil
¼ cup honey
1 egg
1 cup whole-wheat flour
½ cup mashed potato flakes
3½ to 4½ cups bread flour
1½ teaspoons salt

filling

2 tablespoons melted butter

Mix together:
1 cup brown sugar
4 teaspoons cinnamon

Instructions

1. Read the recipe.

2. Grease two 9x5-inch loaf pans with solid white vegetable shortening. I like to use baking parchment to line the loaf pans when I make cinnamon bread.

3. Pour 1 cup of warm water into a large mixing bowl. Sprinkle 1 tablespoon yeast over the water. Stir until the yeast dissolves.

4. Add 1 cup slightly warm milk, ¼ cup light olive oil, ¼ cup honey and 1 egg to the yeast mixture. Stir.

5. In the flour bin, before measuring the flour, sift through the flour with a fork. Spoon the flour into the cup and level with the straight side of a knife.

6. Add 1 cup whole-wheat flour, ½ cup potato flakes, 1½ cups bread flour and 1 and ½ teaspoons salt to the yeast mixture. Stir.

7. Gradually add 2 cups bread flour, stirring with a spoon. The dough will stick together and pull away from the sides and bottom of the bowl. If the dough does not pull away from the sides and bottom of the bowl, add a little more flour until it does. The dough forms a lump.

8. Preheat the oven to 350 degrees.

9. Measure 1 more cup bread flour. Only use what is necessary to knead and shape the dough. Lightly dust the work surface with flour. Place the dough on the work surface. Lightly dust the dough with flour and begin to knead.

10. As you knead, continue to lightly dust the work surface and the dough with flour, so the dough does not get sticky. Knead the dough for about 5 minutes, until it is smooth and elastic.

11. Cut the dough into 2 equal pieces. Shape each piece into a ball. Let the 2 balls rest on the work surface for 5 minutes before shaping them.

12. Keep the work surface and the dough lightly floured. Pat the first ball out into a rectangle, about 6x15-inches, using your hand and a rolling pin. The exact size does not matter.

13. Melt 2 tablespoons butter.

14. Brush the dough lightly with 1 tablespoon melted butter. Leave a ½-inch border all the way around the dough without the butter.

15. Sprinkle the buttered area of the dough with ½ of the cinnamon mixture. Spread it out evenly with your hand.

16. Starting with the 6-inch side nearest you, firmly roll the dough away from you into a log. Pinch the seam together and push into the loaf. Push in and tuck under the two ends of the loaf. Place in the loaf pan seam down and adjust the shape, so the loaf is uniform. Repeat with the second ball.

17. Let the loaves rise until double in size, a process that usually takes about 10 to 15 minutes. Place the loaves into the oven.

18. Bake the loaves for 35 to 40 minutes or until golden brown on the top, sides and bottom. Cinnamon bread needs to cook a little longer than other loaf bread, so the center will not be raw. Check the loaves halfway through the baking time. Rotate the pans in the middle of the baking time for more even baking.

19. Immediately take the loaves out of the bread pans and cool them on a wire cooling rack. The loaves need to cool for 20 minutes before cutting them.

20. When the bread is cool, slice it on a breadboard with a serrated knife. Use a sawing motion as you cut, so you do not squash the bread.

21. Give thanks. Eat some. Share some.

22. Write notes on the recipe, if you make any changes.

Variations

Follow all the steps for cinnamon bread except where new directions are given.

Cinnamon/Raisin Bread

15. Sprinkle the buttered area of the dough with ½ of the cinnamon mixture. Spread it out evenly with your hand.

    Sprinkle ½ cup raisins on the cinnamon mixture before you roll up the dough. If the raisins are hard, first soak them in hot water for 5 minutes and drain them well. Dry them with a paper towel before adding them to the dough. Repeat with the second ball.

ROLLS

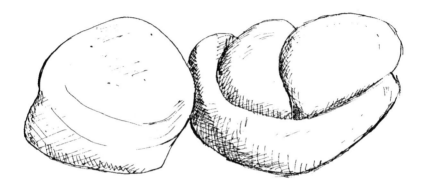

Italian Rolls

These are delicious white rolls that can be made as dinner rolls or made larger for hamburger buns.

Yield

10 large rolls or 12 medium rolls

Ingredients

1 cup warm water
1 tablespoon instant yeast
1 tablespoon and 2 teaspoons granulated sugar
¼ cup light olive oil
1 egg
2¾ to 3¾ cups flour
1 teaspoon salt

glaze

1 beaten egg

As you stay focused on making the bread, your mind will quiet. Enjoy the peacefulness.

Instructions

1. First read the recipe. If you need more help, read the Techniques section.

2. Cover the baking sheet with a piece of baking parchment or grease the baking sheet with solid white vegetable shortening.

3. Pour 1 cup of warm water into a large mixing bowl. Sprinkle 1 tablespoon yeast over the water. Stir until the yeast dissolves.

4. Add 1 tablespoon and 2 teaspoons granulated sugar, ¼ cup light olive oil and 1 egg to the yeast mixture. Stir until well blended.

5. In the flour bin, before measuring the flour, sift through the flour several times with a fork.

Use a serving spoon to scoop the flour into the measuring cup, until it is overflowing. Then with the straight side of a knife, remove the excess flour so that the flour is level with the top of the cup. Measure any type of flour this way.

6. Add 1¾ cups bread flour and 1 teaspoon salt to the yeast mixture. Stir until the mixture is thick and smooth.

7. Add 1 cup bread flour, stirring with the spoon. The dough will stick together and pull away from the sides and bottom of the bowl. If the dough does not pull away from the sides and bottom of the bowl, add a little more flour until it does. The dough forms a lump.

8. Preheat the oven to 350 degrees.

9. Measure 1 more cup bread flour. Only use what is necessary to knead and shape the dough. Lightly dust the work surface with flour. Place the dough on the work surface. Lightly dust the dough with flour and begin to knead. Roll dough should feel softer than bread dough.

10. As you knead, continue to lightly dust the work surface and the dough with flour, so the dough does not get sticky. Knead the dough for about 5 minutes, until it is smooth and elastic.

11. Cut the dough into 10 to 12 equal pieces. Let the pieces rest on the work surface for 5 minutes before shaping them.

12. Keep the work surface and the dough lightly floured. Shape each piece into a ball with the smoothest part as the outside of the ball and place the balls on the baking sheet. If you need help with how to shape rolls, see Shape in the Techniques section.

13. Let the rolls rise until double in size, a process that usually takes about 10 to 15 minutes.

14. Brush the tops of the rolls with beaten egg. Place the rolls into the oven.

15. Bake the rolls for 18 to 22 minutes or until golden brown on the tops and bottoms. Check the rolls halfway through the baking time. Rotate the baking sheet in the middle of the baking time for more even baking.

16. When the rolls have finished baking, take the rolls off the baking sheet with a pancake turner and place them on a wire cooling rack. Rolls can be eaten warm.

17. Give thanks. Eat some. Share some.

18. Write notes on the recipe about the amount of bread flour you used, the rising time, the baking temperature, the baking time and any changes you made to the recipe. If things did not go well, read the section; Things That Can Go Wrong and How to Fix Them.

19. In a couple of days, make this recipe again. Practice will teach you to make excellent bread.

Variations

Follow all the steps for Italian rolls except where new directions are given.

Milk Rolls

3. Pour ½ cup warm water into a large mixing bowl. Sprinkle 1 tablespoon yeast over the water. Stir until the yeast dissolves. Add ½ cup slightly warm milk. Stir.

Buttermilk Rolls

3. Pour ½ cup of warm water into a large mixing bowl. Sprinkle 1 tablespoon yeast over the water. Stir until the yeast dissolves. Add ½ cup slightly warm buttermilk. Stir.

Whole-wheat Rolls

4. Add ¼ cup honey, ¼ cup light olive oil and 1 egg to the yeast mixture. Stir.

6. Add ½ cup whole-wheat flour, 1¼ cups bread flour and 1 teaspoon salt to the yeast mixture. Stir until the mixture is thick and smooth.

Oat Rolls

4. Add ¼ cup honey, ¼ cup light olive oil and 1 egg to the yeast mixture. Stir.

6. Add ¾ oat flour, 1 cup bread flour and 1 teaspoon salt to the yeast mixture. Stir until the mixture is thick and smooth.

Cinnamon Rolls

Soft, light, wonderful. Everyone enjoys them.

Yield

12 rolls

Ingredients

1 cup warm water
1 tablespoon instant yeast
¼ cup melted butter
½ cup slightly warm milk
¼ cup honey
1 egg
1 cup whole-wheat flour
1¾ to 2¾ cups bread flour
1 teaspoon salt

filling

1 tablespoon melted butter

Mix together:
½ cup brown sugar mixed with 1½ teaspoons of cinnamon

glaze

¾ cup powdered sugar
1 tablespoon melted butter
1 tablespoon soft cream cheese
1 teaspoon vanilla or almond flavoring
1 to 2 tablespoons milk

Instructions

1. Read the recipe.

2. Cover the baking sheet with a piece of baking parchment or grease the baking sheet with solid white vegetable shortening.

3. Pour ½ cup of warm water into a medium size bowl. Sprinkle 1 tablespoon yeast over the water. Stir until the yeast dissolves.

4. Melt ¼ cup butter in a sauce pan. Let the butter cool. Add ½ cup slightly warm milk, ¼ cup honey and 1 egg. Stir. Add to the yeast mixture. Stir.

5. In the flour bin, before measuring the flour, sift through the flour with a fork. Spoon the flour into the cup and level with the straight side of a knife.

6. Add 1 cup whole-wheat flour, ¾ cup bread flour and 1 teaspoon salt to the yeast mixture. Stir.

7. Gradually add 1 cup bread flour, stirring with the spoon. The dough will stick together and pull away from the sides and bottom of the bowl. If the dough does not pull away from the sides and bottom of the bowl, add a little more flour until it does.

8. Preheat the oven to 350 degrees.

9. Measure 1 more cup bread flour. Only use what is necessary to knead and shape the dough. Lightly dust the work surface with flour. Place the dough on the work surface. Lightly dust the dough with flour and begin to knead. Roll dough should feel softer than bread dough.

10. As you knead, continue to lightly dust the work surface and the dough with flour, so the dough does not get sticky. Knead the dough for about 5 minutes, until it is smooth and elastic.

11. Shape the dough into a ball. Let the ball rest on the work surface for 5 minutes.

12. On a lightly floured work surface, using your hands and a rolling pin, roll the ball into a 12x20-inch rectangle.

13. Spread 1 tablespoon melted butter on the rectangle.

14. Sprinkle the cinnamon mixture on top of the butter.

15. Beginning with the 20-inch side nearest you, roll the dough up tightly, jelly-roll style away from you. Pinch the last of the roll firmly to the rolled up dough.

16. Using the serrated bread knife and a sawing motion, cut into 12 rolls. Place on the baking sheet.

17. Let the rolls rise until double in size, a process that usually takes about 10 to 15 minutes. Place rolls in the oven.

18. Bake the rolls for 18 to 22 minutes or until golden brown on the tops and bottoms. Check the rolls halfway through the baking time. Rotate the baking sheet in the middle of the baking time for more even baking.

19. When the rolls have finished baking, use a pancake turner to take the rolls off the baking sheet and place on a wire cooling rack.

20. In a small bowl, mix together ¾ cup powdered sugar, 1 tablespoon melted butter, 1 tablespoon soft cream cheese, 1 teaspoon vanilla and 1 to 2 tablespoons milk. Stir until well blended. The mixture should be thick, but still runny. Add more milk if necessary. Drizzle over warm rolls. Rolls can be eaten warm.

21. Give thanks. Eat some. Share some.

Variations

Follow all the steps for cinnamon rolls except where new directions are given.

Cinnamon/Raisin Rolls

14. Sprinkle cinnamon mixture on top of the melted butter. Sprinkle 1 cup of soft raisins over the cinnamon mixture, before rolling up the dough. If necessary, soften the raisins by soaking them in hot water for 10 minutes. Drain them well and pat the raisins dry with a paper towel, before adding them.

Cinnamon/Apple Rolls

14. Sprinkle the cinnamon mixture on top of the melted butter.

    Sprinkle 1 cup of chopped, peeled apple over the cinnamon mixture, before rolling up the dough.

Soft Pan Rolls

Great butter flavor.

Yield

12 pan rolls

Ingredients

½ cup water
1 tablespoon instant yeast
1 tablespoon honey
¼ cup butter (½ stick butter)
½ cup slightly warm milk
1 egg
¼ cup instant mashed potato flakes
2½ to 3½ cups bread flour
1 teaspoon salt

glaze

2 tablespoons melted butter

Instructions

1. Read the recipe.

2. Grease a 9x13-inch pan.

3. Pour ½ cup of warm water into medium size bowl. Sprinkle 1 tablespoon yeast over the water. Stir until the yeast dissolves.

4. Melt ¼ cup butter in a sauce pan. Let the butter cool. Add ½ cup slightly warm milk, 1 tablespoon honey and 1 egg to the butter. Stir. Add to the yeast mixture. Stir.

5. In the flour bin, before measuring the flour, sift through the flour with a fork. Spoon the flour into the cup and level with the straight side of a knife.

6. Add ¼ cup potato flakes, 1½ cups bread flour and 1 teaspoon salt to the yeast mixture. Stir until the mixture is thick and smooth.

7. Add 1 cup bread flour, stirring with the spoon. The dough will stick together and pull away from the sides and bottom of the bowl. If the dough does not pull away from the sides and bottom of the bowl, add a little more flour until it does. The dough forms a lump.

8. Preheat the oven to 350 degrees.

9. Measure 1 more cup bread flour. Only use what is necessary to knead and shape the dough. Lightly dust the work surface with flour. Place the dough on the work surface. Lightly dust the dough with flour and begin to knead. Roll dough should feel softer than bread dough.

10. As you knead, continue to lightly dust the work surface and the dough with flour. Knead the dough for about 5 minutes until it is smooth and elastic.

11. Cut the dough into 12 pieces. Let the pieces rest on the work surface for 5 minutes before shaping them.

12. Keep the work surface and the dough lightly floured. Shape each piece into a ball with the smoothest part as the outside of the ball and place the balls into the pan 3 across and 4 down.

13. Let the rolls rise until double in size. Brush the top of the rolls with melted butter.

14. Place the rolls in the oven.

15. Bake the rolls for 20 to 25 minutes or until golden brown on the tops and bottoms. Check the rolls halfway through the baking time. Rotate the pan in the middle of the baking time for more even baking.

16. When the rolls have finished baking, let them sit in the pan for 2 to 3 minutes and then gently turn them out on the wire cooling rack. The rolls will be upside down. Gently turn them over. Rolls can be eaten warm. Pull the rolls apart to serve.

17. Give thanks. Eat some. Share some.

Variations

Follow all the steps for soft pan rolls except where new directions are given.

Orange Rolls

3. Pour ½ cup of warm water into a medium size bowl. Stir. Sprinkle 1 tablespoon yeast over the water. Stir until the yeast dissolves.

4. Melt ¼ cup butter in a sauce pan. Let the butter cool. Add ¼ cup milk, ¼ cup orange juice, ¼ cup honey and 1 egg. Stir. Add to the yeast mixture.

   Glaze rolls with a mixture of 1 tablespoon melted butter, 1 cup powdered sugar and 1 to 2 tablespoons orange juice.

PRETZELS

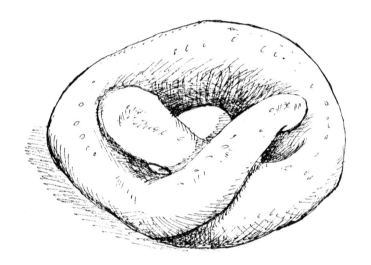

Pretzels

Of all the bread I have ever made, pretzels are the all-time favorite. This recipe makes a firm, chewy pretzel that is very filling and has no oil. They are good cut in half horizontally and toasted. They can be used for sandwiches. The dough can be formed into shapes such as letters, numbers, animals, hearts, etc. This is fun baking activity for kids.

Yield

6 large pretzels or 8 medium sized pretzels

Ingredients

1½ cups warm water
1 tablespoon instant yeast
1 tablespoon honey
½ cup whole-wheat flour
2¼ to 3¼ cups bread flour
1 teaspoon salt

glaze

1 beaten egg for glaze

toppings

coarse salt-sprinkle lightly
or
Parmesan cheese-sprinkle generously
or
poppy seeds-sprinkle as many or few as you wish
or
sesame seeds-sprinkle as many or few as you wish

As you stay focused on making the bread, your mind will quiet. Enjoy the peacefulness.

Instructions

1. First read the recipe. If you need more help, read the Techniques section.

2. Cover the baking sheet with a piece of baking parchment or grease the baking sheet with solid white vegetable shortening.

3. Pour 1½ cups warm water into a large mixing bowl. Sprinkle 1 tablespoon yeast over the water. Stir until the yeast dissolves.

4. Add 1 tablespoon honey. Stir.

5. In the flour bin, before measuring the flour, sift through the flour several times with a fork.

    Use a serving spoon to scoop the flour into the measuring cup, until it is overflowing. Then with the straight side of a knife, remove the excess flour so that the flour is level with the top of the cup. Measure any type of flour this way.

6. Add ½ cup whole-wheat flour, 1¼ cups bread flour and 1 teaspoon of salt to the yeast mixture. Stir until the mixture is thick and smooth.

7. Add 1 cup of bread flour, stirring with the spoon. The dough will stick together and pull away from the sides and bottom of the bowl. If the dough does not pull away from the sides and bottom of the bowl, add a little more flour until it does. The dough forms a lump.

8. Preheat the oven to 400 degrees.

9. Measure 1 more cup bread flour. Only use what is necessary to knead and shape the dough. Lightly dust the work surface with flour. Place the dough on the work surface. Lightly dust the dough with flour and begin to knead

10. As you knead, continue to lightly dust the work surface and the dough with flour, so the dough does not get sticky. Knead the dough for about 5 minutes, until it is smooth and elastic.

11. Cut the dough into 6 to 8 pieces. Shape each piece into a ball with the smoothest part as the outside of the ball. Let the pieces rest for 2 to 3 minutes.

12. Keep the work surface and the dough lightly floured. Choose the smoothest part of the dough as the outside. Roll one piece of dough at a time into a 16-inch rope and form it into the pretzel shape as shown in the drawing. If the work surface is too slippery, brush the flour to the side, lightly grease the work surface with a little solid white vegetable shortening and lightly flour it again. The dough should adhere a little to the work surface, but not stick to it. Place pretzels on the baking sheet pan, leaving room between pretzels.

13. Brush the tops of the pretzels with the beaten egg.

14. Sprinkle on coarse salt, Parmesan cheese, poppy seeds, sesame seeds, or any combination of these.

15. **Pretzels do not rise before putting them in the oven.** Place the baking sheet in the middle of your oven, on the middle rack. Bake the pretzels for 18 to 22 minutes or until golden brown on the tops and bottoms. Check the pretzels halfway through the baking time. Rotate the baking sheet in the middle of the baking time for more even baking.

16. When the pretzels have finished baking, use a pancake turner to take them off the baking sheet and place them on the wire cooling rack. Allow the pretzels to cool for at least 5 minutes.

17. Give thanks. Eat some. Share some.

18. Write notes on the recipe about the amount of bread flour you used, the rising time, the baking temperature, how long it took to bake and any changes to the recipe. If things did not go well, read the section; Things That Can Go Wrong and How to Fix Them.

    Pretzels should be stored in a paper bag, rather than a plastic bag.

    Pretzels get stale quickly because there is no oil in them. Whatever will not be eaten in the first two days should be stored in the freezer.

19. In a couple of days, make this recipe again. Practice will teach you to make excellent bread.

Variations

Follow all the steps for pretzels except where new directions are given.

Whole-wheat Pretzels

6. Add 1½ cups whole-wheat flour and 1 teaspoon of salt to the yeast mixture. Stir until the mixture is thick and smooth.

7. Add 1 cup whole-wheat flour, stirring with the spoon. The dough will stick together and pull away from the sides and bottom of the bowl. If the dough does not pull away from the sides and bottom of the bowl, add a little more flour until it does. The dough forms a lump.

8. Measure 1 more cup of whole-wheat flour. Only use what is necessary to knead and shape the dough. Lightly dust the work surface with flour. Place the dough on the work surface. Lightly dust the dough with flour.

Rye Pretzels

6. Add 1 cup rye flour, ½ cup whole-wheat flour, 1 tablespoon caraway seeds and 1 teaspoon salt to the yeast mixture. Stir until the mixture is thick and smooth.

Cornmeal Pretzels

6. Add ¼ cup cornmeal, 1½ cups bread flour and 1 teaspoon of salt to the yeast mixture. Stir until the mixture is thick and smooth.

Semolina Pretzels

6. Add ¼ cup semolina flour, 1½ cups bread flour and 1 teaspoon salt to the yeast mixture. Stir until the mixture is thick and smooth.

Buckwheat/Fennel Pretzels

6. Add ¼ cup buckwheat flour, 1½ cups bread flour, 1 tablespoon fennel seeds and 1 teaspoon salt to the yeast mixture. Stir until the mixture is thick and smooth.

Pizza/Feta Cheese Pretzels

14. Spread 2 tablespoons of pizza sauce or tomato and basil sauce on top of each pretzel. Sprinkle some crumbled feta cheese on top of the sauce.

Onion Pretzels

14. Mince ¼ cup yellow onion. Sprinkle the minced onion on top of the pretzels.

Garlic Pretzels

14. Mince 2 large garlic cloves. Sprinkle the minced garlic on top of the pretzels.

Everything Pretzels

14. Sprinkle minced garlic, minced onion, poppy seeds, sesame seeds and Parmesan cheese on top of the pretzels.

Pumpkin/Date Pretzels

3. Pour 1 cup warm water into a large mixing bowl. Sprinkle 1 tablespoon yeast over the water. Stir until the yeast dissolves. Add ½ cup canned, mashed pumpkin. Stir.

6. Add ¼ cup whole-wheat flour, 1¼ cups bread flour, 1 teaspoon of salt and ½ cup dates to the yeast mixture. Stir until the mixture is thick and smooth.

Sweet Potato/Cheddar

3. Pour 1 cup of warm water into a large mixing bowl. Sprinkle 1 tablespoon yeast over the water. Stir until the yeast dissolves. Add ½ cup canned, mashed sweet potato. Stir.

6. Add ¼ cup whole-wheat flour, 1¼ cups bread flour, 1 teaspoon salt and ½ cup grated cheddar cheese to the yeast mixture. Stir until the mixture is thick and smooth.

Banana/Macadamia Nut Pretzels

3. Pour 1 cup of warm water into a large mixing bowl. Sprinkle 1 tablespoon yeast over the water. Stir until the yeast dissolves. Add ½ cup mashed banana. Stir.

6. Add ¼ cup whole-wheat flour, 1¼ cups bread flour, 1 teaspoon salt and ½ cup chopped macadamia nuts to the yeast mixture. Stir until the mixture is thick and smooth.

Apple/Cinnamon Pretzels

4. Add 2 tablespoons honey. Stir.

6. Add ¼ cup whole-wheat flour, 1½ cups bread flour, 1 teaspoon salt, ½ teaspoon cinnamon and ½ cup peeled, diced apple to the yeast mixture. Stir until the mixture is thick and smooth.

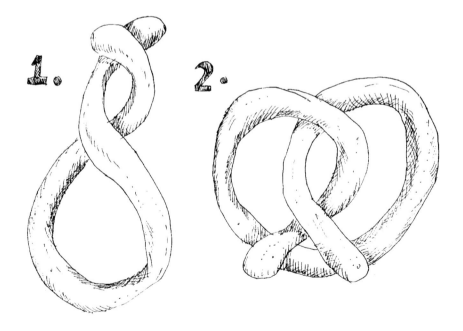

SPECIAL BREAD

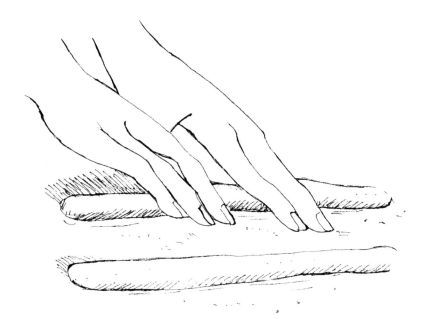

Bread Sticks

Delicious and simple to make.

Yield

8 bread sticks

Ingredients

1½ cups warm water
1 tablespoon instant yeast
1 tablespoon powdered malt or brown sugar
½ cup whole-wheat flour
2¼ to 3¼ cups bread flour
1 teaspoons salt

glaze

1 beaten egg

toppings

Sprinkle on Parmesan cheese
or
rock salt, sesame seeds and poppy seeds
or
glaze with 1 tablespoon melted butter and sprinkle with garlic salt or Parmesan cheese
or
during the last 5 minutes of baking, paint the bread sticks again with the egg mixture and then sprinkle the bread sticks with a little grated cheddar cheese.

As you stay focused on making the bread, your mind will quiet. Enjoy the peacefulness.

Instructions

1. First read the recipe. If you need more help, read the Techniques section.

2. Cover the baking sheet with a piece of baking parchment or grease the baking sheet with solid white vegetable shortening.

3. Pour 1½ cups warm water into a large mixing bowl. Sprinkle 1 tablespoon yeast over the water. Stir until the yeast dissolves.

4. Add 1 tablespoon malt or brown sugar to the yeast mixture. Stir.

5. In the flour bin, before measuring the flour, sift through the flour several times with a fork.

   Use a serving spoon to scoop the flour into the measuring cup, until it is overflowing. Then with the straight side of a knife, remove the excess flour so that the flour is level with the top of the cup. Measure any type of flour this way.

6. Add ½ cup whole-wheat flour, 1¼ cups bread flour and 1 teaspoon salt to the yeast mixture. Stir until the mixture is thick and smooth.

7. Add 1 cup bread flour, stirring with the spoon. The dough will stick together and pull away from the sides and bottom of the bowl. If the dough does not pull away from the sides and bottom of the bowl, add a little more flour until it does. The dough forms a lump.

8. Preheat the oven to 400 degrees.

9. Measure 1 more cup bread flour. Only use what is necessary to knead and shape the dough. Lightly dust the work surface with flour. Place the dough on the work surface. Lightly dust the dough with flour and begin to knead

10. As you knead, continue to lightly dust the work surface and the dough with flour, so the dough does not get sticky. Knead the dough for about 5 minutes, until it is smooth and elastic.

11. Cut the dough into 6 to 8 pieces. Shape each piece into a ball with the smoothest part as the outside of the ball. Let the pieces rest for 2 to 3 minutes.

12. Keep the work surface and the dough lightly floured. Roll one piece of dough at a time into a 9-inch rope. If the work surface is too slippery, brush the flour to the side, lightly grease the work surface with a little solid white vegetable shortening and lightly flour the work surface again. The dough

should adhere a little to the work surface, but not stick to it. Place on a greased or baking parchment covered baking sheet, leaving room between the bread sticks.

13. Brush tops with an egg, beaten with 1 tablespoon water.

14. Choose from the suggested toppings.

15. **Bread sticks do not rise before putting them in the oven.** Place the baking sheet in the middle of your oven, on the middle rack. Bake the bread sticks for 18 to 22 minutes or until golden brown on the tops and bottoms. Check the bread sticks halfway through the baking time. Rotate the baking sheet in the middle of the baking time for more even baking.

16. When the bread sticks have finished baking, use a pancake turner to take the bread sticks off the baking sheet and place them on the wire cooling rack. Allow them to cool for at least 5 minutes.

17. Give thanks. Eat some. Share some.

18. Write notes on the recipe about the amount of bread flour you used, the rising time, the baking temperature, how long it took to bake and any changes to the recipe. If things did not go well read the section; Things That Can Go Wrong and How to Fix Them.

    Bread sticks should be stored at room temperature in a paper bag, rather than a plastic bag.

    Bread sticks get stale quickly because there is no oil in them. Whatever will not be eaten in the first two days should be stored in the freezer.

19. In a couple of days, make this recipe again. Practice will teach you to make excellent bread.

Pizza Dough

Great chewy crust.

Yield

1 large pizza

Ingredients

1½ cups warm water
1 tablespoon instant yeast
1 tablespoon honey
1 tablespoon light olive oil
½ cup whole-wheat flour
2¼ to 3¼ cups bread flour
1 teaspoon salt
3 tablespoons of corn meal for sprinkling the baking sheet

Instructions

1. Read the recipe.

2. Generously rub light olive oil on the baking sheet. Sprinkle the sheet with the 3 tablespoons cornmeal.

3. Pour 1½ cups warm water into a large mixing bowl. Sprinkle 1 tablespoon yeast over the water. Stir until the yeast dissolves.

4. Add 1 tablespoon honey and 1 tablespoon light olive oil to the yeast mixture. Stir.

5. In the flour bin, before measuring the flour, sift through the flour with a fork. Spoon the flour into the cup and level with the straight side of a knife.

6. Add ½ cup whole-wheat flour, 1¼ cups bread flour and 1 teaspoon salt to the yeast mixture. Stir.

7. Add 1 cup bread flour, stirring with the spoon. The dough will stick together and pull away from the sides and bottom of the bowl. If the dough does not pull away from the sides and bottom of the bowl, add a little more flour until it does.

8. Preheat the oven to 425 degrees.

9. Measure 1 more cup bread flour. Only use what is necessary to knead and shape the dough. Lightly dust the work surface with flour. Place the dough on the work surface. Lightly dust the dough with flour and begin to knead. The dough should be soft since you will stretch it into the pan.

10. As you knead, continue to lightly dust the work surface and the dough with flour, so the dough does not get sticky. Knead the dough for about 5 minutes.

11. Shape the dough into a ball. Let the ball rest on the work surface for 10 minutes. Cover with a damp cloth.

12. Oil your hands. Stretch the dough to fit the oiled baking sheet and top with your favorite sauce and topping.

13. Place the baking sheet in the middle of your oven rack, on the lowest rack. Bake the pizza for 20 to 30 minutes until the crust is golden brown. Rotate the baking sheet in the middle of the baking time for more even baking.

14. Slice. Give thanks. Serve hot from the pan.

One of our family's favorite pizza recipes is to spread the dough lightly with tomato sauce. Sprinkle the sauce with Italian seasoning and garlic salt. Then sprinkle with some mozzarella cheese and Parmesan cheese. Top with chopped red, yellow or orange bell peppers, broccoli, purple onion, tomato and olives. Bake.

Focaccia

The best!

Yield

one 12-inch round foccacia

Ingredients

1 cup warm water
1 tablespoon instant yeast
½ cup slightly warm milk
2 tablespoons light olive oil
1 tablespoon honey
1 teaspoon salt
½ cup whole-wheat flour
2¼ to 3¼ cups bread flour
½ cup sliced black olives. Drain olives. Pat olives dry in a paper towel.

1 tablespoon light olive oil to drizzle over the top of the focaccia

Instructions

1. Read the recipe.

2. Cover the baking sheet with a piece of baking parchment or grease the baking sheet with solid white vegetable shortening.

3. Pour 1 cup warm water into a large mixing bowl. Sprinkle 1 tablespoon yeast over the water. Stir until the yeast dissolves.

4. Add ½ cup slightly warm milk, 1 tablespoon honey, and 1 tablespoon light olive oil to the yeast mixture. Stir.

5. In the flour bin, before measuring the flour, sift through the flour with a fork. Spoon the flour into the cup and level with the straight side of a knife.

6. Add ½ cup whole-wheat flour, 1¼ cups bread flour, 1 teaspoon salt and ½ cup sliced black olives to the yeast mixture. Stir.

7. Add 1 cup bread flour, stirring with the spoon. The dough will stick together and pull away from the sides and bottom of the bowl. If the dough does not pull away from the sides and bottom of the bowl, add a little more flour until it does.

8. Preheat the oven to 425 degrees.

9. Measure 1 more cup bread flour. Only use what is necessary to knead and shape the dough. Lightly dust the work surface with flour. Place the dough on the work surface. Lightly dust the dough with flour and begin to knead

10. As you knead, continue to lightly dust the work surface and the dough with flour, so the dough does not get sticky. Knead the dough for about 5 minutes.

11. Shape the dough into a ball. Let the ball rest on the work surface for 10 minutes. Cover with a damp cloth.

12. Place the dough on the baking sheet. Pat with your hands or roll the dough with a rolling pin into a 12-inch round. Let the dough sit for 5 minutes. With your finger, make several indentions in the dough, about 1-inch apart.

13. Drizzle 1 tablespoon light olive oil over the top of the dough.

14. Place the baking sheet in the middle of your oven rack, on the lowest rack. Bake the focaccia for 20 to 30 minutes until the crust is golden brown. Rotate the baking sheet in the middle of the baking time for more even baking.

15. Slice. Give thanks. Serve hot from the pan.

Variations

Follow all the steps for foccacia, except where new directions are given.

Sun-Dried Tomato Focaccia

6. Add ½ cup whole-wheat flour, 1¼ cups bread flour, 1 teaspoon salt and ½ cup sliced sun-dried tomatoes to the yeast mixture. Pat the sun-dried tomatoes dry before adding them to the dough, if they are packed in oil. Stir until the mixture is thick and smooth.

MUFFINS

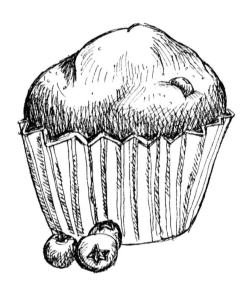

Tips for Excellent Muffins

Use unbleached all-purpose flour, instead of bread flour. The high gluten content in the bread flour will make the muffins tough. Unbleached all-purpose flour has less gluten.

Whole-wheat flour can be substituted for the unbleached all-purpose flour, but the muffins will not be as light.

In one bowl mix the dry ingredients with a spoon or your hands until well blended. It is important that the leavener and salt are equally distributed through-out the dry ingredients. Make sure there are no lumps of baking powder or baking soda. If there are, mash them between your fingers, until they are fine particles.

In another bowl beat the wet ingredients with a whisk or fork until well blended and frothy.

Make a well by pushing the dry ingredients up around the sides of the bowl with a spoon. Pour the wet ingredients into the well. Gently fold the dry ingredients into the wet ones, until all the dry ingredients are moistened. Use only about 15 strokes. The batter may be lumpy. Do not over mix.

Use the 2½-inch muffin cup pans for standard size muffins and the 3¼-inch muffin cup pan for large muffins. The batter will make 12 standard size muffins or 6 large muffins. Spoon batter into the muffin cups. Fill muffin cups two-thirds full. All muffin recipes can also be baked in an 8x8-inch square pan for about 30 minutes.

Bake muffins at 350 degrees for approximately 18 to 20 minutes. Large muffins will need to cook 5 to 10 minutes longer. Check your oven temperature with an oven thermometer to be sure the temperature inside is accurate. Adjust if necessary. Muffins should be baked on the middle rack of your oven, in the middle of the oven. Rotate the pan in the middle of the baking time for more even baking.

Do not open the oven door during the first 10 minutes of baking.

Muffins are done when the tops are lightly browned, the centers are firm to the touch. Do not overbake the muffins or they will be hard.

Let muffins cool for 5 minutes on the wire cooling rack, before removing from the muffin tin. Allow muffins with berries to cool for 10 minutes before removing from the muffin tin. Place the muffins on a wire cooling rack to continue cooling.

Muffins are best served freshly made and slightly warm.

Muffins that you are not going to use within the first 2 days should be frozen.

Muffins must be completely cooled before freezing them. Wrap the muffins tightly in plastic wrap and then place in a plastic freezer zip-lock bag. Try to get the air out of the bag before closing it. Write the date on the bag with a permanent marker. Muffins can be kept in the freezer for 3 months.

To defrost, remove the plastic bag and plastic wrap. Shake off any ice particles. Place on a kitchen towel and allow muffins to defrost at room temperature. An individual muffin can be wrapped in a paper towel and defrosted in a microwave oven for 20 seconds for a standard size muffin and 25 seconds for a large muffin.

Things that Can Go Wrong and How to Fix Them

The muffins are tough.

Did you use bread flour? Bread flour has more gluten in it and will make the muffins tough. Use unbleached all-purpose flour.

Perhaps you stirred the batter too long. The batter should be gently folded, only until the dry ingredients are mixed with the wet. It is all right to have lumps. Use about 15 folding strokes.

The muffins are too heavy.

Did you measure the flour correctly as explained in the recipe? Maybe you added too much flour. Try adding ¼ cup less flour.

Parts of the muffin have a bitter taste.

The baking powder or baking soda was not distributed evenly in the dry ingredients. Make sure the baking powder or baking soda is not lumpy in the dry ingredients or you will taste little bits of it.

Bluberry Muffins

These delicious muffins are loaded with berries. Blueberries add fiber and many important nutrients.

Yield

12 standard size muffins or 6 large muffins

Ingredients

dry ingredients

1 cup unbleached all-purpose flour
¾ cup whole-wheat flour
½ cup brown sugar
2 teaspoons baking powder
¼ teaspoon salt
1½ cups fresh or frozen blueberries

wet ingredients

1 egg
¼ cup light olive oil
1 cup milk

As you stay focused on making the bread, your mind will quiet. Enjoy the peacefulness.

Instructions

1. Read the recipe. If you need more help, read Tips for Excellent Muffins.

2. Preheat oven to 350 degrees.

3. Line muffin cups with foil liners or grease them with solid white vegetable shortening.

4. In the flour bin, before measuring the flour, sift through the flour several times with a fork. If the flour is packed together, you will get too much flour in each cup.

Use a serving spoon to scoop the flour into the measuring cup, until it is overflowing. Then with the straight side of a knife, remove the excess flour so that the flour is level with the top of the cup. Measure any type of flour used in this same way.

5. In a medium size bowl, mix together 1 cup unbleached all-purpose flour, ¾ cup whole-wheat flour, ½ cup brown sugar, 2 teaspoons baking powder and ¼ teaspoon salt, until evenly blended. I like to use my hands to do this. Add 1½ cups blueberries. Stir.

6. In another medium size bowl, add 1 egg, ¼ cup light olive oil and 1 cup milk. Beat together with a whisk or a fork, until well blended.

7. Make a well by pushing the dry ingredients up around the sides of the bowl with a spoon. Pour the wet ingredients into the well. Gently fold the dry ingredients into the wet ones, until all the dry ingredients are moistened. Use only about 15 strokes. The batter may be lumpy. Do not over mix.

8. Using a spoon, fill the muffin cups two thirds full. Place the muffins into the oven.

9. Bake the muffins for 18 to 20 minutes, until the middle of the muffins feel firm to the touch. Rotate the pan in the middle of the baking time for more even baking. Do not over-bake.

10. While still in the muffin tin, let the muffins cool for about 10 minutes on the wire cooling rack. Then remove the muffins from the muffin tin and place them on the wire cooling rack to continue cooling.

11. Give thanks. Eat some. Share some.

Variations

Follow all the steps for blueberry muffins except where new directions are given.

Raisin/Nut Muffins

5. In a medium size bowl, mix together 1 cup unbleached all-purpose flour, ¾ cup whole-wheat flour, ½ cup brown sugar, 2 teaspoons baking powder and ¼ teaspoon salt, until evenly blended. Add 1 cup soft raisins and ½ cup chopped nuts. Stir.

Date Muffins

5. In a medium size bowl, mix together 1 cup unbleached all-purpose flour, ¾ cup whole-wheat flour, ½ cup brown sugar, 2 teaspoons baking powder and ¼ teaspoon salt, until evenly blended. Add 1 cup chopped dates. Stir.

Cheese Muffins

5. In a medium size bowl, mix together 1 cup unbleached all-purpose flour, ¾ cup whole-wheat flour, ¼ cup brown sugar, 2 teaspoons baking powder and ¼ teaspoon salt, until evenly blended. Add 1 cup grated cheese. Stir.

Corn Muffins

Everyone enjoys the flavor of cornmeal.

Yield

6 large or 12 regular muffins

Ingredients

dry ingredients

1 cup unbleached all-purpose flour
½ cup whole-wheat flour
½ cup cornmeal
¼ cup brown sugar
2 teaspoons baking powder
¼ teaspoon salt

wet ingredients

2 eggs
¼ cup light olive oil
¾ cup milk

Instructions

1. Read the recipe.

2. Preheat oven to 350 degrees.

3. Line muffin cups with foil liners or grease them with solid white vegetable shortening.

4. In the flour bin, before measuring the flour, sift through the flour with a fork. Spoon the flour into the cup and level with the straight side of a knife.

5. In a medium size bowl, mix together 1 cup unbleached all-purpose flour, ½ cup whole-wheat flour, ½ cup cornmeal, ¼ cup brown sugar, 2 teaspoons baking powder and ¼ teaspoon salt, until evenly blended. I like to use my hands to do this.

6. In another medium size bowl, add 2 eggs, ¼ cup light olive oil and ¾ cup milk Beat together with a whisk or fork, until well blended.

7. Make a well by pushing the dry ingredients up around the sides of the bowl with a spoon. Pour the wet ingredients into the well. Gently fold the dry ingredients into the wet ones, until all the dry ingredients are moistened. Use only about 15 strokes. The batter may be lumpy. Do not over mix.

8. Using a spoon, fill the muffin cups two thirds full. Place the muffins into the oven.

9. Bake the muffins for 18 to 20 minutes, until the middle of the muffins feel firm to the touch. Rotate the pan in the middle of the baking time for more even baking. Do not over-bake.

10. While still in the muffin tin, let the muffins cool for 5 minutes on the wire cooling rack. Then remove the muffins from the muffin tin and place them on the wire cooling rack to continue cooling.

11. Give thanks. Eat some. Share some.

Variations

Follow all the steps for corn muffins except where new directions are given.

Corn/Bluberry Muffins

5. In a medium size bowl, mix together 1 cup unbleached all-purpose flour, ½ cup whole-wheat flour, ½ cup cornmeal, ¼ cup brown sugar, 2 teaspoons baking powder and ¼ teaspoon salt, until evenly blended. Add 1 cup fresh or frozen bluberries. Stir.

Corn/Cheese Muffins

5. In a medium size bowl, mix together 1 cup unbleached all-purpose flour, ½ cup whole-wheat flour, ½ cup cornmeal, ¼ cup brown sugar, 2 teaspoons baking powder and ¼ teaspoon salt, until evenly blended. Add 1 cup grated cheddar cheese. Stir.

Pumpkin Muffins

I love these pumpkin muffins.

Yield

6 large or 12 regular muffins

Ingredients

dry ingredients

1 cup unbleached all-purpose flour
1 cup whole-wheat flour
½ cup brown sugar
2 teaspoons baking powder
¼ teaspoon salt
1½ teaspoons pumpkin pie spice
1 cup dates

wet ingredients

1 cup canned pumpkin
¾ cup milk
1 egg
¼ cup light olive oil

Instructions

1. Read the recipe.

2. Preheat oven to 350 degrees.

3. Line muffin cups with foil liners or grease them with solid white vegetable shortening.

4. In the flour bin, before measuring the flour, sift through the flour with a fork. Spoon the flour into the cup and level with the straight side of a knife.

5. In a medium size bowl, mix together 1 cup unbleached all-purpose flour, 1 cup whole-wheat flour, ½ cup brown sugar, 2 teaspoons baking powder, ¼

teaspoon salt and 1½ teaspoons pumpkin pie spice, until evenly blended. I like to use my hands to do this. Add 1 cup dates. Stir.

6. In another medium size bowl, add 1 cup canned pumpkin, ¾ cup milk, 1 egg and ¼ cup light olive oil Beat together with a whisk or fork, until well blended.

7. Make a well by pushing the dry ingredients up around the sides of the bowl with a spoon. Pour the wet ingredients into the well. Gently fold the dry ingredients into the wet ones, until all the dry ingredients are moistened. Use only about 15 strokes. The batter may be lumpy. Do not over mix.

8. Using a spoon, fill the muffin cups two thirds full. Place the muffins into the oven.

9. Bake the muffins for 18 to 20 minutes, until the middle of the muffins feel firm to the touch. Rotate the pan in the middle of the baking time for more even baking. Do not over-bake.

10. While still in the muffin tin, let the muffins cool for about 5 minutes on the wire cooling rack. Then remove the muffins from the muffin tin and place them on the wire cooling rack to continue cooling.

11. Give thanks. Eat some. Share some.

Variations

Follow all the steps for pumpkin muffins except where new directions are given.

Banana Muffins

5. In a medium size bowl, mix together 1 cup unbleached all-purpose flour, 1 cup whole-wheat flour, ½ cup brown sugar, 2 teaspoons baking powder and ¼ teaspoon salt until evenly blended. Add ½ cup chopped pecans. Stir.

6. In another medium size bowl, add 1 cup mashed banana, ¾ cup milk, 1 egg and ¼ cup light olive oil Beat together until well blended with a whisk or fork.

Applesauce Muffins

5. In a medium size bowl, mix together, 1 cup unbleached all-purpose flour, 1 cup whole-wheat flour, ½ cup brown sugar, 2 teaspoons baking powder, 1 teaspoon cinnamon, ¼ teaspoon nutmeg and ¼ teaspoon salt until evenly blended. Add ½ cup chopped pecans. Stir.

6. In another medium size bowl, add 1 cup applesauce, ¾ cup milk, 1 egg and ¼ cup light olive oil Beat together until well blended with a whisk or fork.

Bran Muffins

A good source of fiber.

Yield

12 standard size muffins or 6 large muffins

Ingredients

dry ingredients

1½ cups whole-wheat flour
½ wheat bran
½ cup brown sugar
2 teaspoons baking powder
¼ teaspoon salt
½ cup grated carrots
½ cup raisins

wet ingredients

1 egg
¼ cup light olive oil
1 cup milk

Instructions

1. Read the recipe.

2. Preheat oven to 350 degrees.

3. Line muffin cups with foil liners or grease them with solid white vegetable shortening.

4. In the flour bin, before measuring the flour, sift through the flour with a fork. Spoon the flour into the cup and level with the straight side of a knife.

5. In a medium size bowl, mix together 1½ cups whole-wheat flour, ½ cup wheat bran, ½ cup brown sugar, 2 teaspoons baking powder and ¼ teaspoon

salt until evenly blended. I like to use my hands to do this. Add ½ cup grated carrots and ½ cup raisins. Stir.

6. In another medium size bowl, add 1 egg, ¼ light olive oil and 1 cup milk. Beat together with a whisk or a fork, until well blended.

7. Make a well by pushing the dry ingredients up around the sides of the bowl with a spoon. Pour the wet ingredients into the well. Gently fold the dry ingredients into the wet ones, until all the dry ingredients are moistened. Use only about 15 strokes. The batter may be lumpy. Do not over mix.

8. Using a spoon, fill the muffin cups two thirds full. Place the muffins into the oven.

9. Bake the muffins for 18 to 20 minutes, until the middle of the muffins feel firm to the touch. Rotate the pan in the middle of the baking time for more even baking. Do not over-bake.

10. While still in the muffin tin, let the muffins cool for about 5 minutes on the wire cooling rack. Then remove the muffins from the muffin tin and place them on the wire cooling rack to continue cooling.

11. Give thanks. Eat some. Share some.

Gingerbread

Moist and delicious.

Yield

8x8-inch square pan
12 pieces

Ingredients

dry ingredients

1 cup whole-wheat flour
½ cup unbleached all-purpose flour
1 teaspoon baking soda
1 teaspoon powdered ginger
½ teaspoon cinnamon
¼ teaspoon allspice
¼ teaspoon salt

wet ingredients

½ cup buttermilk
½ cup molasses
1 egg
¼ cup light olive oil

Instructions

1. Read the recipe.

2. Preheat oven to 350 degrees.

3. Grease and flour or line the baking pan with baking parchment.

4. In the flour bin, before measuring the flour, sift through the flour with a fork. Spoon the flour into the cup and level with the straight side of a knife.

5. In a medium size bowl, mix together 1 cup whole-wheat flour, ½ cup unbleached all-purpose flour, 1 teaspoon baking soda, 1 teaspoon powdered

ginger, ½ teaspoon cinnamon, ¼ teaspoon allspice and ¼ teaspoon salt until evenly blended. I like to use my hands to do this.

6. In another medium size bowl, add ½ cup buttermilk, ½ cup molasses, 1 egg and ¼ cup light olive oil together. Beat together with a whisk or a fork, until well blended.

7. Add the wet ingredients to the dry ingredients and stir untill evenly blended.

8. Spoon the batter into the baking pan.

9. Place the gingerbread into the oven. Bake for 30 to 35 minutes until a toothpick put into the middle come out clean and the middle feels firm to the touch. Rotate the pan in the middle of the baking time for more even baking. Do not over-bake.

10. Let the gingerbread cool for about 10 minutes in the pan on the wire cooling rack. Remove the gingerbread from the pan and place it on the wire cooling rack for further cooling. Slice.

11. Give thanks. Eat some. Share some.

Oatcakes

Very hearty. A good source of energy.

Yield

8x8-inch square pan
12 oatcakes

Ingredients

dry ingredients

1½ cups whole-wheat flour
¾ cup brown sugar
1 teaspoon baking soda
¼ teaspoon salt
3 cups oatmeal
1 cup chopped dates
½ cup diced dried cherries
½ cup diced dried apricots

wet ingredients

1 cup plus 2 tablespoons soymilk
1 egg
1 teaspoons vanilla
2 tablespoons light olive oil

Instructions

1. Read the recipe.

2. Preheat oven to 350 degrees.

3. Grease and flour or line the baking pan with baking parchment.

4. In the flour bin, before measuring the flour, sift through the flour with a fork. Spoon the flour into the cup and level with the straight side of a knife.

5. In a medium sized bowl, mix 1½ cups whole-wheat flour ¾ cup brown sugar, 1 teaspoon baking soda and ¼ teaspoon salt until evenly blended. I like to use my hands to do this. Add 3 cups oatmeal, 1 cup chopped dates, ½ cup diced dried cherries, and ½ cup diced dried apricots. Stir.

6. In another medium bowl, add 1 cup, plus 2 tablespoons soymilk, 1 egg, 1 teaspoon vanilla and 2 tablespoons light olive oil. Beat together with a whisk or a fork, until well blended.

7. Pour the wet ingredients into the dry ingredients. Mix them all together, using your hands.

8. Push the batter into the pan. It will be very dense. Flatten.

9. Place the oatcakes into the oven. Bake the oatcakes for about 30 minutes until firm and slightly browned. Rotate the pan in the middle of the baking time for more even baking.

10. Remove from the pan to a wire cooling rack. Remove the baking parchment from the cake.

11. When cooled, cut into 12 squares.

12. Give thanks. Eat some. Share some.

Variations

Follow all the steps for oatcakes except where new directions are given.

5. Use different dried fruits than the ones in the recipe. Add nuts.

6. In a medium bowl, beat 1 cup plus 2 tablespoons milk, 1 egg, 1 teaspoon vanilla and 2 tablespoons light olive oil together with a whisk or fork.

Glossary

boil: to heat a liquid until bubbles rise to the surface and break.

dissolve: to turn a solid ingredient into a liquid ingredient.

dough: a dense uncooked mixture of liquid, flour and yeast.

drizzle: to drip a glaze from the end of the spoon over rolls.

dusting: to lightly sprinkle flour on a work surface so the dough will not stick to it.

elasticity: the ability of the dough to stretch and rise.

fiber: the roughage of the grain.

fold: to gently lift and turn over the dry ingredients into the wet ingredients until all the dry ingredients have been moistened.

glaze: to paint a liquid topping onto the bread or rolls before or after they are baked.

greasing: to rub fat on the pan to prevent sticking.

humidity: the amount of water in the air.

leaven: that which makes the dough or batter rise such as yeast, baking powder or baking soda.

mince: to cut into very small pieces.

oven spring: the dough rises higher in the oven.

rising: the process of the dough growing bigger.

stir: to combine ingredients with a spoon or whisk using a circular motion.

stone ground: coarsely ground wheat.

yield: the amount the recipe will make.

"The Bosom Buddies of Hawaii program is a service provided to women with breast cancer diagnosis, for up to one year. It is free of charge. Each woman is matched with a Healing Touch practitioner, her Bosom Buddy, who will offer her Healing Touch treatments.

The client and her Bosom Buddies volunteer meet regularly, working together to promote healing and self-care. Clients experience results ranging from increased relaxation and pain relief to enhanced recovery after surgery.

Bosom Buddies of Hawaii is housed at The Queen's Medical Center in Honolulu (www.queens.org) and is sponsored by a dozen organizations in Hawaii, including the American Cancer Society."

A donation from the sale of each book will be given to Bosom Buddies of Hawaii. (www.bosombuddieshi.org)

BIBLIOGRAPHY

Brown, Edward Espe, *The Tassajara Bread Book*. Boston: Shambhala Publications, Inc. 1986.

Casella, Dolores. *A World of Bread*. Port Washington, New York: David White, Inc. 1996.

Hensperger, Beth, *The Bread Bible*. California: Chronicle Books. 1999.

Pillsbury Publications, *The Complete Book of Baking*. New York: Viking Penguin. 1993

Reinhart, Peter. *Brother Juniper's Bread Book: Slow Rise As Method and Metaphor*. Addison-Wesley Publishing Company. 1991.

ORDERING INFORMATION

Contact iUniverse

Call: toll-free: 877-823-9235

Or call: Kathy Summers: 808-263-4570

0-595-30451-6